EPISIOTOMY AND THE SECOND STAGE OF LABOR

Episiotomy and the Second Stage of Labor

Edited by
Sheila Kitzinger
and for North America
Penny Simkin

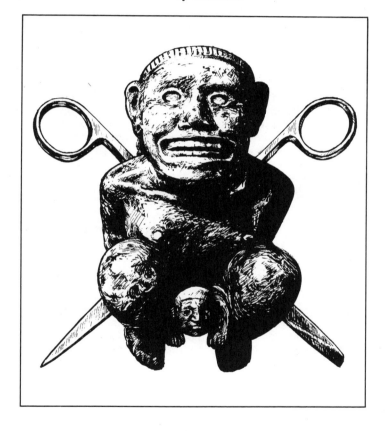

Second Edition

pennypress, inc.

Chapter 2 was first published in the Journal of Obstetrics and Gynaecology of the British Commonwealth 64(6):815-820, 1957, and is reprinted here with permission.

Chapter 4 was first published in Kaleidoscope of Childbearing: Preparation, Birth and Nurturing, edited by Penny Simkin and Carla Reinke. Seattle: Pennypress, 1978. Reproduced here with permission.

Chapters 6, 10, and 11 were previously published in Episiotomy: Physical and Emotional Aspects, edited by Sheila Kitzinger. London: National Childbirth Trust, 1981. Reproduced with permission.

Chapter 9 was first published in the Birth and the Family Journal 9(1):25-30, Spring 1982, and is reprinted here with permission.

*   *   *   *   *   *   *   *

The cover art is a drawing of an ancient Aztec sculpture of the Goddess, Tlazoltéotl, giving birth in a squatting position.   The primitive stone sculpture, with the surgical steel scissors, illustrate two contrasting approaches to the second stage of labor.

Cover illustration by Terry Furchgott
Illustrations for Chapter 11 by Angela Owen
Book design by Tom Lenon
Index for Second Edition by Kay Heeren, MSLS

Library of Congress Number   84 - 61122
ISBN 0-937604-07-0 paperback

Table of Contents

Preface and Acknowledgements

Episiotomy and the Second Stage of Labor began as a North American edition of Episiotomy: Physical and Emotional Aspects, edited by Sheila Kitzinger and published by the National Childbirth Trust in the United Kingdom. The National Childbirth Trust granted North American publishing rights to Pennypress, Inc. But as the book was being prepared for publication, it became evident to publisher Penny Simkin that the differences between British and North American episiotomy practices were so great that the book would need to be changed and expanded for application in North America. Some of those differences are:

* Most births in North America are attended by obstetricians or family practitioners -- very few by midwives; in the United Kingdom, most births are attended by midwives or general practitioners.
* Midline episiotomy is the rule in North America; mediolateral episiotomy is the rule in the United Kingdom.
* All birth attendants in North America can do both episiotomies and their repair; in the United Kingdom midwives can do episiotomies but many are not allowed to do the repair. Women therefore sometimes have a long waiting period before their episiotomies are repaired.
* Medical care in the United States is a part of the American economic system of free enterprise. Patients pay for their care; economic incentives exist for physicians to have busy practices and to use time-saving measures and money-making procedures. This is balanced somewhat by economic incentives to please their patients who are more able and more likely to shop carefully for a physician or to change physicians if they do not like what they are paying for. Canada's system of socialized medicine is similar to that in the United Kingdom.

It is not clear exactly how these differences affect maternity care, but it is obvious that the two systems are not interchangeable, and findings in one system may not be easily applied to the other.

Therefore, the book underwent vast changes. Only three of the chapters in Episiotomy: Physical and Emotional Aspects remain essentially unchanged. Nine chapters and four appendices have been added to alter and expand the scope of the book to cover second stage management generally, as well as the subject of episiotomy.

We wanted to retain and even expand the outstanding contributions of experts from countries outside North America, in an effort to apply their knowledge to North American practices. We also have reprinted here several highly significant papers which we felt help to complete the discussion of the topic.

The editors wish to thank the National Childbirth Trust for their generosity in granting publication rights, and the contributors to this book, not only for their papers, but also for their concern for childbearing families that led them to the work presented here. We also wish to thank Fran Cihon and Jane Hatfield of Pennypress: Fran for cheerfully, carefully and tirelessly typing and retyping the manuscripts; Jane for competently maintaining the day-to-day business operations, allowing preparation of the book to continue.

Preface to the Second Edition

We were gratified by the interest shown in the first edition of <u>Episiotomy and the Second Stage of Labor,</u> and decided to reprint it with minor revisions and two major additions: Chapter 13, a review of recent research findings; and an author and subject index.

We wish to thank Kay Heeren for proofreading the text and preparing the indexes -- jobs requiring the utmost in patience and attention to detail. We are also grateful to secretary Cynthia Nelson and typist Caroline Simkin for their care in making the manuscript corrections and additions.

Introduction

Sheila Kitzinger

Episiotomy is the most commonly performed obstetric operation. It is the only surgery likely to be performed without her consent on the body of a healthy woman in Western society.

Although midwives in England used to try to avoid episiotomy unless there was evidence that the perineal tissues were not fanning out well, it is now an accepted part of a normal delivery. Its use has increased steadily in England over the past 15 or 20 years, while remaining extremely high in North America ever since the 1930s.

The rise in the rate of episiotomy is one side-effect of the move from home to hospital birth, from individual responsibility to "team" obstetrics and from the control of childbirth by the mother or midwife to its control by the obstetrician. In North America, where midwifery has never been accepted as the model for maternity care, the obstetrical model with its greater use of intervention of all kinds has prevailed.

The National Childbirth Trust (N.C.T.) conducted a survey of 1795 women who had attended their classes in England and Wales during a definite period and who had vaginal deliveries. Of these, 65% had episiotomies, 20% had lacerations, and only 15% had no injury to the perineum. They reported some disturbing findings[1]:

    * Although 40% of respondents found suturing painless and almost as many that it was "bearable," 23% said it was "painful" or "very painful."

    * By the end of the first week after delivery, 67% felt the perineal area was comfortable or mildly uncomfortable, but 32% were still in pain.

    * The majority of women never discussed the issue of episiotomy with a doctor or midwife during pregnancy. Thirty-seven percent of those who had an episiotomy were never given a reason for it and of the 62% who had some explanation, many were told after, rather than before, it was performed. Whereas 15% of those who knew the reason had forceps deliveries and understood that the episiotomy was to allow room for instruments, 26% of those who had episiotomies were informed simply that they were too small and that it was done to protect against a tear. They were often told "It is better to have a neat cut than a jagged tear," "It is easier for the doctor to sew up," "It is done so that you don't get prolapse in

middle age," or sometimes "If you don't have an episiotomy you won't be able to enjoy intercourse later."

* It was not uncommon for a woman to have a tear as well as an episiotomy. Nine percent of women knew they had had both. There were probably more of which women were unaware.

* Episiotomy is often performed rather soon in the second stage. There may be good clinical reasons for this, but it may also be a matter of an unquestioned routine procedure. In many hospitals partograms are used; slower than average progress in expulsion is an indication for obstetric intervention. The second stage may have a time limit, for some obstetricians it is two hours, for others one and a half hours, one hour, forty-five minutes or even half an hour. The midwife receives instructions to call the obstetrician if labor continues beyond this limit. As a result midwives often perform episiotomies to avoid calling the doctor, since this will usually result in a forceps delivery. Thus, even if in practice it is frequently the midwife who performs the episiotomy, she does so as part of the management of labor controlled by the obstetrician. In the N.C.T. survey episiotomy was performed in the first half hour of the second stage in 44% of cases and before three quarters of an hour were up in 62% of cases. An episiotomy done early on a thick perineum increases the risk of heavy bleeding, because the time between episiotomy and delivery is prolonged.

* Episiotomy may also sometimes be performed when not strictly necessary as part of the training of both medical students and student midwives. Occasionally medical students who have previously stitched only a cut finger in casualty, are required to suture as soon as they arrive in the delivery suite and are inadequately supervised as they do so.

* Painful suturing, stitches which are too tight and which allow no room for the inevitable swelling following injury, stitches which fall out before they are supposed to, leaving distended tissues, a gaping hole or a flap of skin, absorbable sutures which fail to be absorbed and which become deeply embedded in skin, perineal infection and granulation of scar tissue are all frequently described.

Many women would endure this willingly if they believed it helped their babies. In fact, they are often told that an episiotomy is performed for the baby's sake. Yet in spite of claims that episiotomy makes birth safer for the baby, there have been no studies comparing the outcome for the infant in episiotomy and no-episiotomy groups. Episiotomy certainly speeds delivery and it is often taken for granted that a rapid second stage must be better for the baby. Research, however, suggests that the length of the second stage per se does not harm the healthy fetus.[2]

The evidence for the routine or liberal use of episiotomy is unconvincing. Episiotomy is an example of an intervention which has been introduced into obstetric practice without accurate assessment and without asking women what they prefer.

We hope that these papers will be of assistance to those working in midwifery, obstetrics and gynecology, to antenatal teachers wishing to help women learn how they can help themselves, those faced with the task of counselling mothers suffering postpartum sexual difficulties, and to all women who want to have choice in childbirth.

REFERENCES

1. Kitzinger S. and Walters R. Some Women's Experiences of Episiotomy. London, National Childbirth Trust, 1981.

2. Butler N.R., Alberman E.D. (eds.), Prenatal Problems. London, Livingstone, 1960.

INTRODUCTION

Penny Simkin

The popular American textbook, Williams Obstetrics, devotes no space to a consideration of indications for episiotomy or its risks, nor to methods of protecting the perineum and avoiding episiotomy or tears.

Questions of appropriateness of episiotomy are dismissed by Pritchard and MacDonald as follows: "It can be said with certainty that, since the era of in-hospital deliveries with episiotomy, there has been an appreciable decrease in the number of women subsequently hospitalized for treatment of symptomatic cystocele, rectocele, uterine prolapse, and stress incontinence!"[1] There are no references supporting this enthusiastic endorsement, and in fact, no studies have been done of long-term effects of episiotomy versus non-episiotomy.

Any questions regarding episiotomy center on: when in second stage episiotomy should be performed; whether it should be a median or mediolateral incision; whether repair should be done before or after the placenta is expelled; and which suture materials and repair techniques to employ. Such unquestioning approval of the routine use of episiotomy deters impressionable medical students and young physicians from a healthy questioning of a fundamentally radical, painful and potentially risky surgical procedure.

While North America probably leads the world in its acceptance of routine episiotomy, in the last decade we have seen and heard women protesting what they interpret as a thoughtless disregard for this highly sensuous and sexual part of their bodies. Episiotomy is surgical injury, frequently followed by pain, poor healing and dyspareunia. Alternatives to the procedure exist, but they require patience, manual skills and a commitment to preserving the perineum intact or, if that is not possible, to doing minimal damage and repairing it skilfully.

When the issue of episiotomy is raised, its proponents usually state that there must be a choice between fetal well-being and preservation of the maternal perineum. They point out that episiotomy benefits the baby and that avoiding it compromises the fetus, who is traumatized by passing through the birth canal.

In fact, the evidence presented in this book suggests *management of second stage to protect the perineum from episiotomy or tearing is also management to protect fetal well-being.* Such management combines several features which together serve to protect both mother and fetus:

1. Maternal positioning for comfort, progress, and avoidance of stress on the perineum, also protects the fetus from the secondary effects of supine hypotension and reduces the need for forceps.

2. Spontaneous (short and intermittent) maternal bearing-down efforts alternated with breathing stretch perineal tissues more gradually than prolonged breathholding and straining, and also allow for better fetal oxygenation.

3. Perineal massage and support, hot compresses, and low-key encouragement for spontaneous bearing down, enhance gradual stretching of the vagina while avoiding the emotionally stressful "crisis" atmosphere usually present during delivery where the woman is exhorted to push the baby out as fast as possible. Such stress itself, by causing the outpouring of catecholamines, can result in poor fetal oxygenation.

Therefore, proponents of such conservative management believe it is rarely necessary to make a choice between the fetus and the mother.

In this book an international panel of experts from various childbirth-related fields examines all aspects of second stage management, especially episiotomy. We hope the book will influence second stage management practices and reduce the episiotomy rate to the benefit of women and their babies.

On a personal note, I would like to dedicate this book to my parents, Thomas and Caroline Payson, who taught me through example and conscious guidance that what seems to be is not necessarily what is.

REFERENCES

1. Pritchard J.A. and MacDonald P.C. <u>Williams Obstetrics</u>, 16th edition. New York, Appleton-Century-Crofts, 1980: p. 430.

1. Active and Physiologic Management of Second Stage: A Review and Hypothesis.

Penny Simkin, R.P.T.

Second stage management has evolved over the past 65 years without the benefit of controlled prospective clinical trials. Here an American childbirth educator and student of the obstetrical literature traces this evolution of management practices and describes the objections raised along the way. She also presents a physiologic model for understanding and managing the normal second stage.

The basic principles guiding management of the second stage of labor were established during the 1920s and have remained virtually unchanged and largely unquestioned since. Many of the conventional wisdoms (guiding labor management) ". . . although not based on fact, . . . had been relayed from teacher to student, and textbook to textbook, without any serious attempt at critical analysis until they have come to represent possibly the main impediment to progress in this field."[1] The few published reports which raised questions seem to have created a slight stir and then been ignored until recently.[2,3,4] Thus, debate on the basics of management has been sparse, and there has been little change. Major refinements in second stage management have taken place only in such areas as anesthesia, episiotomy techniques, and guidelines for the use of forceps, vacuum extractor and cesarean section.

In this paper I will describe both active and physiologic management of the second stage and the reasoning that has led to each. I will also describe a model for understanding and interpreting the events of the normal second stage, in hopes of revising the conventional approach to the second stage.

FEATURES OF THE TWO TYPES OF MANAGEMENT

In active management, interventions by the birth attendant are used with the intent of controlling and improving the birth process. In physiologic management, the spontaneous birth process is maintained and encouraged by understanding, supporting and enhancing the body's normal mechanisms of birth.

On the one hand interference in the spontaneous process is seen as improving it; on the other, interference is seen as carrying unnecessary and potentially harmful side-effects. See Table 1 for a comparison of the features of active and physiologic management.

TABLE I: SECOND STAGE MANAGEMENT

Features of Active Management	Features of Physiologic Management
Dorsal propped position, then lithotomy for birth.	Any of a number of positions (may try several), and movement.
"Pushing on command" -- prolonged breathholding with maximum bearing down or straining throughout each contraction.	Spontaneous (usually short) bearing down and breathholding as urge demands.
Anesthesia (regional or local block) reduces sensation, urge to push, and muscle tone in perineum.	Sensations (urge to push and burning, stinging) guide mother's efforts.
Anesthesia-induced relaxation of pelvic floor.	Conscious relaxation of pelvic floor.
Mother placed on delivery table with stirrups to enable administration of anesthesia, episiotomy, use of forceps or vacuum extractor.	Mother uses bed, birth chair or stool, beanbag chair, squatting bar, human support, or other.
Sterile field.	Mother encouraged to touch baby's head.
Episiotomy.	Perineal massage & support.
Forceps/vacuum extractor for: fetal distress, lack of progress, maternal exhaustion, approaching time limit, malposition of baby, inability to push effectively.	Combined influences of mother's pelvic floor muscle tone, spontaneous bearing down, contractions, and gravity rotate and bring baby down.

These two approaches are based on very different belief systems. Acceptance of different sets of principles logically leads people to different approaches. Following is a description of the principles guiding active management with a discussion of how these principles came to be so widespread. Later in the paper is a similar description and discussion of physiologic management.

Principles Guiding Active Management of Second Stage

1. Second stage is traumatic to the fetus.
2. The longer the second stage, the poorer the outcome for the baby.
3. Episiotomy benefits the baby by reducing head compression and shortening the second stage.
4. Episiotomy benefits the mother by preventing tears or undue stretching of the perineum.
5. The lithotomy or modified lithotomy position is the preferred position for second stage.

In sum, management techniques are evaluated by their potential for hastening the second stage. Active management became the rule as the result of widespread acceptance of particular assumptions about the second stage, which, although not based on research findings, were forcefully stated and actively promoted by highly respected and well-known obstetricians of the time.

These principles evolved during the late 19th and early 20th centuries, when prevailing circumstances favored a shift to active management: stereotypes of the weakness of women; the emergence of a medical specialty focused on female reproduction; transition of birth from the home to the hospital; middle and upper class women's desires for liberation from the confinement imposed by pregnancy and from the pain of childbirth.

Women were considered to be "inherently frail . . . also predisposed to insanity;"[5] or the "nervous inefficient products of modern civilization."[6] Such attitudes, plus the alarmingly high neonatal and maternal mortality rates of the time, were at least partly responsible for the specialization in obstetrics by physicians. More and more women entered the hospital to have their babies, partly because it was believed to be safe and free from dreaded disease-causing germs, and partly because twilight sleep (a combination of scopolamine and morphine) became available for the relief of childbirth pain.

Concerns that women were constitutionally unfit for normal childbirth were matched by concerns that the fetus was traumatized by passage through the birth canal. Conveniently, physicians saw themselves as benefiting both mothers and babies through widespread use of analgesia and anesthesia, episiotomy and forceps.

Joseph DeLee, a prominent Chicago obstetrician in the first forty years of this century, is credited with laying the groundwork for modern active management. He proposed "eliminating" the second stage by routinely using episiotomy and forceps under general anesthesia. In his classic paper, "The Prophylactic Forceps Operation,"[6] he catalogued the dangers of birth to both mother and baby in expressive prose:

> I have often wondered whether Nature did not deliberately intend women should be used up in the process of reproduction, in a manner analogous to that of the salmon which dies after spawning?[6]

> The fetal brain suffers "prolonged pounding and congestion"[6] in a hard spontaneous delivery, with possible brain damage and anoxemia or asphyxia.

R. H. Pomeroy, another prominent American obstetrician of the time, referred to the child's head during second stage as "a battering ram wherewith to shatter . . . a resisting outlet."[7] This reference to the baby's head as a "battering ram" was resurrected in 1950 in Williams Obstetrics, 10th edition, where it has remained in all six editions since.

Although DeLee's pronouncements prompted debate and were not universally accepted immediately, his method of general anesthetic, episiotomy and forceps soon became the rule. Refinements in anesthesia technique, infection control, indications for forceps vs. cesarean section, and in attitudes toward maternal participation have modified DeLee's approach somewhat, but his underlying principles, based on the dangers of second stage to mother and baby and the desirability of aggressive management to speed or eliminate the second stage, continue to dictate second stage management to a large extent.

Principles Guiding Physiologic Management of Second Stage

1. Second stage benefits the fetus by stimulating the mobilization of energy stores and the secretion of hormones -- catecholamines, prostaglandins, endorphins and others -- which promote extrauterine adaptation.
2. The duration of second stage is better dictated by fetal and maternal condition than by an arbitrary time limit.
3. Spontaneous maternal behavior (short bearing-down efforts alternated with slow or

light rapid breathing) prevents undue compression of the fetal skull by allowing gradual relaxation and stretching of the pelvic floor musculature.

4. Spontaneous maternal behavior in physiologically favorable positions allows for gradual distention of the perineum and little or no damage.

5. Maternal positions for second stage should be selected for their benefits to maternal comfort, fetal well-being or progress in labor. The wide variety of positions selected by women rarely includes lithotomy or supine with knees drawn up toward shoulders.

Principles guiding physiologic management are based on the underlying assumption that the unassisted birth process is usually safe, healthy and beneficial to mother and baby. Medical interventions are reserved for abnormal situations.

Physiologic management is directed toward maintaining maternal comfort, fetal well-being, an intact perineum, and progress in descent. These principles provide the basis for the features of physiologic management listed in Table 1.

The principles of physiologic management began to emerge in North America in the late 1970s, as Americans became more aware of trends in other countries, and as interest flared in out-of-hospital births, midwife-attended births and hospital birthing centers. Concern over the quality of the birth experience for the baby led to the promotion of gentle birth and parent-infant bonding by Frederic Leboyer,[8] Michel Odent,[9] Marshall Klaus and John Kennell.[10] These new emphases in childbirth made it inevitable that many of the "tried-and-true" conventional wisdoms in childbirth education and in labor management would be re-examined. For years Sheila Kitzinger, first in the United Kingdom, later in North America, had been advocating "breathing the baby out"[11] rather than forcefully expelling the baby. Elizabeth Noble[12] and Roberto Caldeyro-Barcia[13] raised important questions regarding the safety of prolonged Val Salva maneuvers to expel the baby. J. G. B. Russell[14] Claudio and Moyses Paciornik,[15] Anna Flynn,[16] Peter Dunn,[4] Carlos Mendez-Bauer and Joyce Roberts[17] described and documented benefits from movement during labor and use of a variety of positions for birth. Dunn[4] and Caldeyro-Barcia[13] revived concerns, first reported more than a decade before, over iatrogenic maternal hypotension and fetal distress caused by the supine position and its resulting compression of the aorta and inferior vena cava. Sheila Kitzinger,[18] David Banta and Stephen Thacker[19] reopened the question of the value and wisdom of widespread use of episiotomy. The relationship between length of second stage and neonatal outcome was questioned by W. R. Cohen[20] and Doris Haire.[21] Several investigators[22,23,24] reported that the indices of fetal well-being relied upon during first stage (fetal heart rate patterns, scalp blood pH) did not apply to the second stage, and that bradycardias first appearing in late second stage are not associated with poor Apgar scores.

While all the rules about second stage were being challenged, midwives and laboring women, quietly giving birth in homes and birthing centers, were breaking every one of them and forming a new approach to the second stage.

Many childbirth educators, dissatisfied with their "cookbook" approach to second stage, were highly receptive to a more physiologic approach and began requesting workshops to learn more about the physiologic approach to the second stage of labor. Manufacturers of birthing beds and chairs began designing their products to facilitate physiologic positioning of laboring women.

Most physicians, midwives, and the maternity nurses working with them, however, continue today using active management, preferring supine, semi-reclining or lithotomy positions, prolonged breathholding and straining, anesthesia and episiotomy, with frequent use of forceps or vacuum extractor.

PROBLEMS WITH ACTIVE MANAGEMENT

The question arises, then, how many of the problems that we associate with second stage are caused, not by the passage of the fetus through a tight space, but by active management itself? Do the alleged advantages gained by active management (speed, control and convenience) justify the disadvantages?

Consider the following: The supine, lithotomy or semi-lithotomy positions offer convenience to the birth attendant, but cause supine hypotension and fetal heart rate decelerations.[4] This position contributes to the "fetal distress" which makes speed of delivery appear necessary.

Prolonged breathholding and straining by the mother throughout each contraction of second stage is intended to speed second stage. That it is effective has not been confirmed scientifically,[25,26] but it is known to be associated with fetal hypoxia[27] and maternal exhaustion, thus also contributing to apparent fetal distress.

Caudal, epidural, and spinal anesthesia, and even pudendal block, all of which provide pain relief and allow for use of forceps if the need arises, actually increase the incidence of forceps deliveries by causing fetal distress secondary to maternal hypotension, slowing labor, impeding the cardinal movements due to profound relaxation of the pelvic floor musculature, and by diminishing the Ferguson reflex (bearing-down reflex) and outpouring of oxytocin which otherwise occur during second stage.[28] In addition, the mother cannot readily change position or bear down as effectively as an unanesthetized woman.

The advantages of episiotomy have long been assumed, but not established scientifically.[19] The risks of episiotomy, and the circumstances under which episiotomy is indicated and not indicated have not been established scientifically. If episiotomy is indicated in cases of fetal distress, there is need to establish what is fetal distress in second stage, and to avoid causing it when possible. If episiotomy is to prevent undue stretching of the perineum, it has to be done early in second stage, before significant stretching has taken place. This increases the risk of hemorrhage, because blood supply to the perineum is generous early in the second stage, diminishing only with compression of blood vessels by the descending head. Since most practitioners believe such risks are not worth taking, it is unlikely that episiotomy, performed as it usually is, late in second stage, prevents undue stretching of the perineum.

Fetal heart rate decelerations during the second stage cause concern and lead to action to hasten the delivery, making fetal distress a common indication for the use of forceps and episiotomy. Even though such decelerations are often the result of the supine position and prolonged Val Salva maneuvers (breathholding and straining), discontinuation of these harmful behaviors is rarely utilized as a way to correct the decelerations. In fact, the mother is usually expected to increase her Val Salva maneuvers, in hopes of further hastening the delivery.

"FETAL DISTRESS" DURING SECOND STAGE

The issue is further complicated by recent findings that fetal heart rate decelerations first appearing during expulsion are not associated with low Apgar scores or poor neonatal condition.[22,23] A healthy fetus apparently has the ability to mobilize sufficient reserves to counteract some oxygen deprivation. Catecholamines or stress hormones are secreted by the fetus when deprived of oxygen, allowing for shunting of blood from non-vital to vital organs, increased extraction of oxygen from available blood, and mobilization of energy stores. The catecholamine response assures that the healthy fetus extracts sufficient oxygen even though there is less oxygenated blood available.[29,30] However, fetuses who have previously been compromised during pregnancy and/or labor may be unable to withstand the added stress of the second stage. Our ability to select them is poor at this time.

Therefore, fetal distress, as presently diagnosed, does not necessarily result in neonatal distress; in fact the correlation between the two is rather poor,[31] leading some investigators to question the prognostic value of a diagnosis of fetal distress.

Such findings leave the clinician in a difficult situation. The very fetuses in greatest need of rapid delivery, besides being difficult to detect, may be least able to tolerate the means for rapid delivery (such as anesthesia, supine position to allow episiotomy and forceps, prolonged straining and breathholding), many of which add to the stress.

Because selection is difficult, clinical protocols tend to assume that all bradycardias are indications of complications requiring immediate delivery. Alternatively, some innovative physicians and midwives, motivated by the preferences of their clients, are utilizing their knowledge of the woman's and fetus' prenatal and intranatal course, preventive measures such as non-supine positions, spontaneous bearing-down, and avoidance of anesthesias associated with maternal hypotension and fetal bradycardias to create optimum conditions for spontaneous birth and an intact perineum.

THE NORMAL SECOND STAGE

Following is a hypothetical model of the normal second stage derived from the writer's observations of normal labors without interventions and behavioral restrictions; also from published descriptions[2,3,32] and anecdotes from midwives, nurses, physicians and recently delivered women. The model provides a framework for integrating, clarifying, and explaining these observations, and provides a rationale for physiologic management.

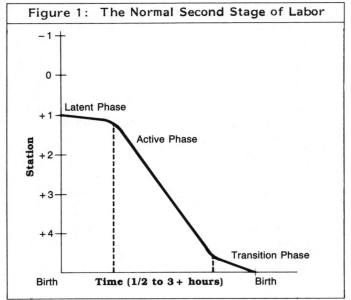

Figure 1: The Normal Second Stage of Labor

Latent Phase
Active Phase
Transition Phase
Station
−1
0
+1
+2
+3
+4
Birth   Time (1/2 to 3 + hours)   Birth

The second stage can be divided into phases, much as the first stage is. During each phase, different work is accomplished, and the mother's emotions, sensations, and spontaneous behavior change. The distinct nature of each phase fades if the station is low (+2 or lower) when the second stage begins.

Friedman described a model of descent similar to the one above, including three phases or periods: latent, acceleration and deceleration.[33] His observations indicated the latent and part of the active periods of descent occur before dilatation is complete and that the average station at onset of second stage is "well beyond the midplane"[34] (+2 or lower station). Frequently, however, station is much higher at the onset of second stage; if so there is likely to be a distinct latent or resting phase experienced during second stage, as indicated in Figure 1.

THE LATENT PHASE

The latent phase of descent, commonly observed after dilatation is complete, is characterized by an apparent decrease in uterine activity. During this phase, which commonly lasts 10 to 20 minutes, the mother gets a chance to rest, collect herself after the intensity and confusion of transition, and look ahead to the birth. The lull in uterine contractions may be due to cervical retraction around the fetal presenting part. As dilatation nears completion, the cervix not only dilates but it begins drawing up (retracting) around the fetal presenting part.[33] When retraction of the cervix has occurred, the presenting part slips out of the uterus. If the presenting part is the fetal head, it represents one fifth to one fourth the surface area of the fetus. When it slips out, the uterus, which had been tightly stretched around the fetus, may be left somewhat "flabby." It takes time for the fibers of the uterus to shorten sufficiently to tighten around the body of the fetus. During this time (the latent phase) uterine activity is not readily apparent, and the mother may notice neither contractions nor an urge to push. The latent phase ends and the active phase begins when the uterus is once again stretched tightly around the fetus, resumes contracting forcefully, the mother feels an urge to push, and the fetus descends.

THE ACTIVE PHASE

During this phase, the strong contractions, combined with periodic bearing-down efforts result in rapid descent, which may or may not be uncomfortable for the mother. Degree of discomfort is associated with fetal position (occiput anterior positions seem to be associated with less pain than transverse or posterior positions), maternal position, elasticity of maternal tissue, and size of the presenting part. Mothers should be encouraged to seek positions of greater comfort at this time; these will often also result in greater progress. If one carefully observes maternal behavior and uterine activity during the active phase of the second stage, it becomes obvious that bearing-down efforts are clearly in response to changes in the uterus.

The urge to push comes and goes during second stage and is clearly tied in with extra "surges" in uterine contractility that occur three to five times during the contractions. Kitzinger describes "surges of desire to bear down," and that only the mother can know when they are there.[35] Caldeyro-Barcia has described such surges but interpreted them somewhat differently.[16] He interpreted the spontaneous bearing-down efforts, with their increase in abdominal muscle tone, as causing the increased intrauterine pressure seen periodically during these active phase second stage contractions. This writer interprets the increases in intrauterine pressure as causing the accompanying bearing-down effort. In other words, even if a woman does not bear down at all, the periodic short increases in intrauterine pressure would occur, except, possibly, when anesthesia is used.

Each surge is thus accompanied by an involuntary bearing-down effort by the mother and obvious progress in descent of the fetus. These surges can often be anticipated if the birth attendant or labor support person places a hand on the fundus. The contraction is clearly felt, and superimposed on the contraction is an additional sudden increase in tonus (the surge) felt as an extra tightening, almost a knotting of the uterus, which lasts 5 to 7 seconds. It then recedes for a few seconds, to reappear several times during the contraction.

If a mother is encouraged to behave spontaneously during the second stage, she breathes during the contractions, except during these surges when she bears down, either with breathholding or with exhalation (grunting, yelling, or straining sounds). The presenting part advances during the surges and retreats between, until the crowning in late second stage, at which time it stops slipping back between bearing-down efforts. This represents the onset of the transition phase of the second stage.

It is during the active phase that a woman needs reassurance, reminders to open up, relax and bulge the perineum, since the alarming sensations of fetal descent may cause her to tense the perineum and "fight" against descent. Hot compresses and perineal massage are also helpful aids.

What the woman does not need at this time are exhortations to "Push! Push! Push!" and a supine position. As has already been stated, such "pushing on command" has not been found to shorten the second stage, and the supine position is known to be inefficient and potentially detrimental to fetal well-being (see Carr and Caldeyro-Barcia chapters in this volume). Spontaneous bearing-down and maternal positioning for comfort and/or progress are preferable.

THE TRANSITION PHASE

It is during the transition phase of the second stage that the fetus emerges -- from crowning to birth of the entire body. The transition phase is thus named because: 1) this phase represents the transition from fetus to neonate, and 2) there are many similarities to the transition phase of the first stage in terms of emotional intensity, confusion and pain. The transition phase is characterized by extreme, sometimes alarming, sensations of burning and stretching of the vagina as the head and perhaps the shoulders are born. The mother may be confused: On the one hand, she is anxious to push hard to get her baby out quickly; on the other, she needs to protect her perineum by easing her baby out.

During the transition phase, which may last one to several contractions, a woman needs reassurance that the burning sensation is normal, and reminders to relax her perineum and to blow rather than push. She need not rush the birth. Hot compresses, perineal massage and support, and the opportunity to touch her baby's head or to watch the birth in a mirror bring comfort and valuable feedback to the woman at this time.

The emotional and physical intensity of the latter part of second stage and its abrupt end may leave a woman needing time to absorb the fact that it is over (or nearly so). She may need a moment to grasp that her body is no longer sending these intense painful signals before she is able to shift her attention to the baby. On the other hand, she may have no emotional pause as she flows through second stage to claim her baby -- touching her baby's head as it descends and emerges, reaching down, drawing the baby from her body to her chest.

IMPLICATIONS FOR MANAGEMENT

The goals of physiologic management of second stage are a healthy vigorous neonate, an emotionally satisfied mother with an intact perineum, and full physical and psychological capabilities to interact with and breastfeed her baby. All this can best be accomplished by maintaining a harmony between the physiologic process, the efforts of the mother, and the efforts of the attending staff.

This harmony begins to be established beforehand, with education. The woman and her partner(s) benefit from learning in advance what to expect during second stage. The following six points need to be well understood as they enter second stage:

1. Anatomical, physiological and emotional events.
2. Explanation of sensations: urge to push, pressure within the vagina, burning and stretching, and variations in these sensations and in pain experienced related to fetal size, station, position and other factors.
3. The many possible positions for second stage and the advantages and disadvantages of each.
4. The value of the pelvic tilt and perineal massage.
5. The importance of relaxation of the pelvic floor (use of imagery, calm verbal support, a mirror, hot compresses and touching the baby's head to help relaxation).
6. The importance of NOT rushing the second stage (avoiding the cheerleading approach, avoiding the word "Push!").

Assuming a healthy pregnancy and a normal first stage of labor, there is no need to rush. The mother need make no efforts to push during the latent phase. She simply needs reassurance and an explanation of what is happening. During the active phase, she is encouraged to yield to the surges in her uterus, bearing down when she must. She is also encouraged to move into positions of comfort and to release her pelvic floor: "Ease the baby out," "Open for the baby," "Relax your bottom." Very hot compresses and perineal support and massage (see Appendix D) may assist her in relaxing and opening.

When she begins feeling the burning and stretching of the transition phase, this is a clear signal to avoid bearing down, so as not to tear. Because it hurts even more to push, she will respond well to calm reminders to avoid bearing down, reassurance that the burning is normal at this time.

MANAGEMENT FOR PROBLEMS IN SECOND STAGE

If it becomes necessary to intervene to enhance progress or to remedy apparent fetal distress, the following general rules of management are a helpful guide:

1. When all is normal, do as little as possible to interfere;

2. If interference becomes desirable, it should first take the form of enhancing the physiologic process: e.g., change of position to enhance relaxation of the perineum, rotation and descent, or to correct fetal heart rate problems; hot compresses and perineal massage; very hard long pushing ("purple pushing").

3. If unsuccessful, then use interventions which replace the physiologic process: e.g., medication, vacuum extractor, forceps, episiotomy.

CONCLUSION

In this chapter we have traced the historical pathway to today's active management; discussed the problems with this approach; documented the development of a newer and more conservative approach to second stage management; provided a model for understanding the normal second stage; and discussed general principles of management.

It should be clear that a physiologic approach is a "package:" a combination of elements (position, bearing-down efforts, conscious maternal participation, comfort measures, support, etc.) which allow the harmonious interaction of numerous critical factors. Denying or replacing part of the package may interfere with the overall process, making total intervention necessary.

REFERENCES

1. O'Driscoll K, Meagher D. Active Management of Labour. London, WB Saunders Company Ltd., 1980: pp. 3-4.

2. Beynon CL. The normal second stage of labour: a plea for reform in its conduct. J Obstet Gynaecol Br Commonw 64(6):815-820, 1957. (Reprinted in this volume.)

3. Read GD. Childbirth Without Fear: The Original Approach to Natural Childbirth. New 4th edition, revised and edited by Wessel H and Ellis HF. New York, Harper & Row, 1972.

4. Dunn PM. Obstetric delivery today: for better or for worse? Lancet I(7963):790-793, 10 April 1976.

5. Rothman SM. Women's Proper Place. New York, Basic Books, Inc., 1978: p. 24.

6. DeLee J. The prophylactic forceps operation. Am J Obstet Gynecol 1:34, 1920.

7. Pomeroy RH. Shall we cut and reconstruct the perineum for every primipara? Am J Obstet Dis Wom Child 78:211-220, 1918.

8. Leboyer F. Birth Without Violence. New York, Knopf Publishing Co., 1975.

9. Odent M. Entering the World: The De-Medicalization of Childbirth. London, Marion Boyars, Inc., 1984. (First published in French in 1976.)

10. Klaus M and Kennell J. Maternal-Infant Bonding. St Louis, CV Mosby Co., 1976.

11. Kitzinger S. The Experience of Childbirth. New York, Taplinger Publishing Co., 1972: p. 129.

12. Noble E. Respiratory considerations in childbirth, in Kaleidoscope of Childbearing - Preparation, Birth and Nurturing, edited by Simkin P and Reinke C. Seattle, Pennypress, 1978.

13. Caldeyro-Barcia R. Influence of maternal bearing-down efforts during second stage on fetal well-being, in Kaleidoscope of Childbearing - Preparation, Birth and Nurturing, edited by Simkin P and Reinke C. Seattle, Pennypress, 1978. (Reprinted in this volume.)

14. Russell JGB. Moulding of the pelvic outlet. J Obstet Gynaecol Br Commonw 76:817-820, Sep 1969.

15. Paciornik C, Paciornik M, and Centeno SP. Implications of the squatting position birth in the mother-child relationship: Experience from 528 cases. Personal communication, 1977.

16. Flynn AM, Kelly J, et al. Ambulation in labour. Br Med J 2:591-593, 26 Aug 78.

17. Roberts JE, Mendez-Bauer C, and Wodell DA. The effects of maternal position on uterine contractility and efficiency. Birth 10(4):243, Winter 83.

18. Kitzinger S and Walters R. Some Women's Experiences of Episiotomy. London, National Childbirth Trust, 1981.

19. Banta D and Thacker S. Benefits and risks of episiotomy: An interpretative review of the English language literature, 1860-1980. Obstet Gynecol Survey 38(6):322-338, Nov 83. (Summary of this paper reprinted in this volume.)

20. Cohen WR. Influence of the duration of second stage labor on perinatal outcome and puerperal morbidity. Obstet Gynecol 49(3):266-269, Mar 77.

21. Haire D. The Cultural Warping of Childbirth. Milwaukee, International Childbirth Education Association, 1972.

22. Katz M, Shani N, et al. Is end-stage deceleration of the fetal heart ominous? Br J Obstet Gynaecol 89(3):186-189, Mar 82.

23. Gaziano EP, Freeman DW, et al. FHR variability and other heart rate observations during second stage labor. Obstet Gynecol 56(1) Jul 80.

24. Ohel G. Fetal heart rate in the second stage of labour and fetal outcome. S Afr Med J 54:1130, 30 Dec 78.

25. Yeates DA and Roberts JE. A comparison of two bearing-down techniques during the second stage of labor. J Nurs Midwif 29(1):3-11, Jan/Feb 84.

26. Barnett MM and Humenick SS. Infant outcome in relation to second stage labor pushing method. Birth 9(4):221-229, Winter 82.

27. Caldeyro-Barcia R, et al. Physiological and psychological bases for the modern and humanized management of normal labor, in Recent Progress in Perinatal Medicine and Prevention of Congenital Anomaly [Editors not stated on the reprint.] Tokyo, Medical Information Services, Inc., 1980.

28. Vasicka A, Kumaresan P, et al. Plasma oxytocin in initiation of labor. Am J Obstet Gynecol 130(3):263-273, 1 Feb 78.

29. Phillippe M. Fetal catecholamines. Am J Obstet Gynecol 146(7):840-855, 1 Aug 83.

30. Jones CM and Greiss FC. The effect of labor on maternal and fetal circulating catecholamines. Am J Obstet Gynecol 144(2):149-153, 15 Sep 82.

31. Steer P. Has the expression 'fetal distress' outlived its usefulness? Br J Obstet Gynaecol 89(9):690, Sep 82.

32. Moore WMO. The conduct of the second stage, in Benefits and Hazards of the New Obstetrics, edited by Chard T and Richards M. Philadelphia, JB Lippincott Co., 1977.

33. Friedman EA. Labor: Clinical Evaluation and Management, 2nd Edition. New York, Appleton-Century-Crofts, 1978.

34. Friedman EA, same as above: p. 42.

35. Kitzinger S. The Complete Book of Pregnancy and Childbirth. New York, Alfred A Knopf, 1980: p. 209.

2. The Normal Second Stage of Labor: A Plea For Reform in its Conduct.

Constance L. Beynon, M.B., F.R.C.S.(Edin.), M.R.C.O.G.

(Reprinted with permission. First appeared in Journal of Obstetrics and Gynaecology of the British Commonwealth 64(6):815-20, 1957.)

The need to rush the second stage predominates in the minds of most birth attendants. In a classic paper reprinted here, a British obstetrician describes spontaneous bearing down by primiparous women, and documents the advantages of such behavior in the preservation of pelvic structures.

Over the past twenty-five years many changes have taken place in the conduct of normal labor. One of the most outstanding features is the elimination of the sense of haste in the first stage. Many practicing today will not remember the older type of midwife who honestly believed that the speedy end of the ordeal was what mattered to the patient rather than its tolerability. She resisted any suggestion of inducing rest and sleep because of its delaying action and morphia she abhorred. This idea has now virtually disappeared and we have achieved an atmosphere of tranquility with relaxation of tension by various means. But this atmosphere is still confined to the first stage; the management of the second stage has changed little over the years; the prevailing note is still one of hard work and making haste. This is clearly reiterated in many standard textbooks. Claye (1955) states "the patient should now be working very hard". Greenhill (1955) in his textbook says "the patient is working hard; the process is indeed labour"; he also mentions the veins of the neck standing out, the face being turgid and the body bathed in sweat. Miles (1956) in a midwives' textbook gives detailed instruction on how to teach and encourage the mothers to push, and illustrates how to extract the maximum of effort from them when required. She does however state that the pushing should not start until the head is showing. Moir (1956) and others also teach reservation of forced straining till the head has reached the pelvic floor. De Soldenhoff (1956) specifically states that relaxation should continue during the early part of the second stage but he too encourages pushing when the head is on the pelvic floor. Many doctors and midwives still seem to consider it their function to aid and abet and even coerce the mother into forcing the fetus as fast as she can through her birth canal.

The question is how much straining is necessary or desirable and when should it be used? The purpose of this paper is to suggest that for most women less straining is required than is practiced today and that the minimum is the optimum.

THE SPONTANEOUS SECOND STAGE

If the mother is left entirely to her own intuition in the second stage several important details can be observed.

1. The amount of voluntary straining is slight until the head begins actively to distend the pelvic floor but thereafter completely involuntary and irresistible straining efforts occur with a mechanism so similar to defecation as to be almost indistinguishable from it.

2. This straining mechanism does not come into play at the onset of each uterine contraction or pain; there is a clear interval between the onset of the contraction and the patient's impulse to exert herself.

3. It is worthy of note that there is often considerable variation in the amount of push behind each pain; some have very little and are short and mild, while others are associated with a strong impulse and great progress.

To demonstrate these features convincingly the patient should have no pre-conceived ideas, nor should she inhibit herself in any way. The second stage usually progresses remarkably well even with heavy sedation and the process can be readily studied in such cases. (This, however, is not to be taken as an advocacy of heavy sedation at this stage of labor.) If the patient who is obviously trying to force the pace can be stopped from pushing altogether for a few pains, and this often requires great persuasion at first, she will usually then fall into the correct rhythm and her better progress and greater ease has to be witnessed to be believed. In practice it has been found necessary to be constantly aware of the tendency in many women toward too early, or too hard pushing. Many patients, it is well known, try to push before full dilatation and insist that they have the urge; we stop them with great conviction. But a considerable number of patients claim to have the urge later who, although fully dilated, will still be much wiser not to push. Jeffcoate (1950) says that it is better to begin expulsive efforts too late than too soon. I would add that it is also better to strain too little than too much.

Two cases are quoted to illustrate these points:
Case 1. Mrs. F. Para-O. Age 24

Many years ago, before I had even contemplated this method, I was asked to go to this patient who was well on in labor and look after her pending the arrival of her own doctor who was delayed at another confinement. My colleague was particularly anxious to be present at this delivery so I resolved to do nothing to hurry the process unless it was necessary. We ignored the patient's early straining efforts and when finally the head reached the pelvic floor, just allowed it to emerge slowly on minimal pushing, hoping every minute that her doctor would walk in. The baby (8 pounds 3 ounces) was born before the doctor arrived but with practically no effort on the part of the patient and an intact vagina and perineum. The peacefulness and obvious ease of the birth were most impressive.

Case 2. Mrs. S. Para-O. Age 32

This was a recent case conducted in a unit which is schooled in minimal pushing. The patient was herself a trained nurse and her obstetrician husband was present. I was called for the delivery and arrived to find the head distending the pelvic floor and the patient exerting herself moderately to expel it. I too thought this was completely spontaneous and irresistible but after watching a few pains and noting the small amount of progress relative to the patient's effort I became doubtful. The perineum was tense and shiny yet I knew this patient had a good outlet and I had thought also that she had good pelvic floor tissues. Episiotomy seemed indicated but acting on my doubts I asked the patient to try very hard to stop pushing altogether for about ten pains. After a few pains without pushing the labor took on a completely different aspect and with very slight but irresistible straining the head oozed out without any vaginal or perineal laceration whatever.

In the first case quoted, the reason for not encouraging pushing was purely social but it is common knowledge that in cases where pushing is undesirable or impossible (as in some paralyses) easy labor is remarkably common. The relative ease of cardiac cases is well recognized. F. J. Browne (1955) quotes a forceps rate of less than 5 per cent in cardiac cases in University College Hospital, when no straining has been allowed and states that this is no higher than the rate for the hospital as a whole. It almost seems that the inability to strain may be an advantage. Theoretical explanations for this will be discussed later.

For many years now I have adopted the practice of allowing my patients to follow their own inclination in the second stage, forbidding all mention of pushing by those in attendance. Sometimes considerable patience is required at the beginning of the expulsive stage but the easier advance later fully compensates for this. Those who have witnessed the method have been impressed by the ease of expulsion of the fetal head and by the tranquil atmosphere which can be achieved, but those who are not familiar with the procedure have often expressed difficulty in believing that the duration of the second stage will not be unduly prolonged or the forceps rate rise. It was therefore decided to conduct an independent clinical trial to see if these doubts were with foundation or not.

CLINICAL TRIAL

This trial was carried out at the Sussex Maternity Hospital by two experienced labor ward sisters previously unfamiliar with the method. Normal primigravidae with vertex presentations were assessed; all such cases booked under me and delivered by day were conducted as below; there was no other selection. One hundred consecutive cases were tested and compared with the total of 393 other normal primigravid vertex deliveries occurring over the same period. The procedure followed was that no suggestion to the patient that she should push was allowed unless the labor was not progressing satisfactorily. No other alteration was made in the routine conduct of the case. If any suggestion was ever necessary the case was recorded as a failure. The results are shown in Figure 1. Of the 100 cases, 83 delivered themselves entirely spontaneously, the average duration of the second stage in them being 1 hour and 3 minutes. One second stage lasted 3 hours but with very infrequent short pains, and one 2 hours and 10 minutes; no others lasted over 2 hours. Fifteen of the 83 babies weighed over 8 pounds, 3 of them being over 9 pounds, and one weighed 10 pounds 9 ounces. Six of the hundred cases ended in forceps delivery despite ultimate encouragement to push, but the forceps rate for the tested cases was still only about half that of the controls (47 of 393 cases = 11.9 per cent). This left only 11 cases who could be said to have shown a need for coercion and in 6 of these the decision that encouragement was required had been reached before the second stage had lasted 2 hours and therefore may have been premature. The suture rate for the group was also less than for the controls: 39 of the 100 required sutures as compared with 63 per cent (249) of the controls. (In calculating these figures episiotomies for whatever indication were included on both sides.)

These results show the effect of conducting the second stage along a pattern which reserves instruction in pushing entirely for those who have proved their need of it. The series was a purely clinical experiment to see if it was possible to refute the idea that labor is of necessity prolonged and the interference rate raised if patients are not taught and encouraged to strain. The sisters conducting the trial, although never advocates of excessive pushing, had not practiced the method before nor had I discussed it at length with them. They were selected purposely for their lack of bias, associated with complete reliability and sound clinical judgment. The method has been discussed and practiced to a considerable extent in other units under my care and those midwives who have worked with me longest and have really schooled themselves in its use have become increasingly convinced of its value.

THEORETICAL CONSIDERATIONS

That an entirely spontaneous second stage is the ideal mode of delivery can I believe be supported by theoretical as well as practical considerations.

There is first the simple principle that slow distension is less traumatic than sudden or rapid stretching and therefore one would expect less laceration of fascial and muscle layers as well as fewer skin or mucosal tears.

The next consideration concerns the supports of the uterus and of the vaginal vault. If the fetus were to be expelled through the lower uterine segment and vagina only by a piston-like or squeezing action of the upper part of the uterus there would be little tendency to a downward thrust of the cervix or adjoining vagina and therefore no dragging on the transverse cervical ligaments or the connective tissue supports of the vaginal vault. In the truly spontaneous second stage this very largely applies; it is only when the head has traversed the whole length of the anterior vagina and posteriorly has reached the pelvic floor that outside forces are brought into play. If instead external force is used while the head is gripped by either cervix or vagina the ring of contact will be pushed down and its supports dragged upon (Fig. 2). Here then is a possible etiological factor in prolapse of the type described by Malpas (1955) as utero-vaginal. That this form of prolapse may result from pushing before full dilatation of the cervix has long been accepted, but the submission here is that it can also apply in some measure to pushing at any time before the head has impinged forcibly on the pelvic floor. Danforth (1947) has shown that in the Rhesus monkey the level of the cervix rises considerably during the second stage of labor reaching its greatest height toward the end of that stage, but in the human the cervical lips have been shown to rise only to the level of the pelvic inlet (Danforth and Ivy, 1949). The explanation put forward by these writers is that the relatively greater strength or reduced elasticity of the transverse cervical ligament in the human prevents the upward movement. It would seem then that there is a potential pull upward sufficient to resist a downward thrust. The degree of harm to the uterine supports resulting from a downward strain would thus depend on four factors: (1) the amount of strain active externally on the uterus; (2) the relative amount of counter-pull exerted by the upward trend of the parts above the ligaments; (3) the amount of pull or push acting internally, which would depend on the tightness of fit between head and passages; (4) the strength of the transverse cervical ligament and neighboring tissues. Elimination of forced straining would favorably affect the first two factors.

The third consideration is in respect of the anterior vaginal wall and supports of the bladder. In a parous woman a roll of vaginal mucosa can frequently be seen being pushed down in front of the head anteriorly (Fig. 3). If the patient can be persuaded to stop pushing for a few pains the roll will disappear, and then with far less straining than before the head will be delivered. This tendency to downward stress of the anterior vaginal wall must be present in a primipara, although to a less obvious degree. It is easy to imagine the shearing strain which can thus be produced between the vaginal mucosa and its deeper attachments, and the potential damage to the underlying tissues. This may well be one etiological factor in the production of stress incontinence, the urethro-vesical junction supports being as it were torn down. Moir (1956) cites the danger of this fold in a discussion on stress incontinence. He advises that it should be pushed up, but it will disappear spontaneously with a few contractions if straining is strictly avoided, in other words if this concept of the truly physiological second stage is upheld. Watson (1924) suggested this stripping down of bladder fascia as a cause of stress incontinence. He related it to the pushing down of the anterior lip of the cervix, but it could equally apply to the upper vagina if it were being pushed down by a tightly fitting presenting part. Malpas, Jeffcoate and Lister (1949) and Kanton, Miller and Dunlap (1949) have demonstrated that the bladder base and the urethro-vesical junction are not normally raised in position as labor progresses but that they rotate forward with the descent of the presenting part so that bladder base and urethra come to be in a straight line. It is suggested nevertheless that the earlier part of each contraction pulls the vagina taut and prevents it and the structures beneath it from being pushed down in front of the presenting part. Until this tightening has taken place it is undesirable that descent of the fetus should occur.

A parallel has been drawn between the birth canal and a coat sleeve; if now we postulate that the sleeve has a potentially loose lining, two further useful parallels can be drawn. First, the slower the arm is thrust down such a sleeve the less is the tendency for the lining to roll out at the wrist. Secondly, if the lining is held firmly at the top during the maneuver the amount of resistance to the descending arm is considerably reduced, and its passage down the sleeve becomes very much easier.

From time to time it has been suggested that routine episiotomy and even forceps delivery prevent prolapse. It is possible that the knowledge that the instrumental delivery is imminent discourages any forced straining and that it is this absence of straining that produces the better results.

Remembering the stress on the uterine and bladder supports there might be a case for forceps delivery in preference to too vigorous pushing when the head is gripped tightly by the birth canal. Such forceps delivery should however utilize the uterine contractions and allow time for the vagina to be drawn taut before each pull is made.

DISCUSSION

If there is no good reason in theory or in practice for hurrying the second stage of labor, why has the habit been prevalent for so long and why does it still persist?

We have in our era progressed toward greater patience in regard to the first stage of labor. We have, also in our era, learned the advantages of a slower and calmer approach to an allied process, namely defecation. Yet we would seem to have failed to carry the same principles to the expulsive stage of labor. No one would deny that more violent effort is sometimes required in defecation but it is acknowledged as the exception rather than the ideal. Just so in labor; if some 4 primigravidae in every 5 require no encouragement to violent exertion and are better left to take their own time, surely we are falsifying the whole process by being so ready to dictate to them. Instead of hurrying our patients and forcing advice on them about pushing whether they need such advice or not, we would be much more usefully engaged in persuading them to take their time and only allowing them to push, and push gently, when the urge is obviously irresistible.

A clear distinction might profitably be made between those labors which are completely normal and those which depart however slightly from that normal. About 80 per cent of primigravid labors and most multiparous labors should come into the first category. These patients are able to deliver themselves instinctively with little more straining than is required in the process of defecation. All other cases should be put in a different category which would include not only cases requiring operative delivery but also those requiring extra straining efforts. The management of the second category must remain a matter for individual discrimination but surely sound obstetric practice should aim primarily at giving every woman a reasonable chance to achieve complete normality.

Many obstetricians and midwives already feel, and some quite strongly, that too much pushing is being encouraged and they are trying to reduce it; some are also trying to eliminate pushing in the second stage until the head has reached the pelvic floor. Not so long ago obstetricians had to make a stand against the habit of an earlier generation of encouraging pushing from the very onset of labor. Everyone now accepts that pushing before full dilatation is both useless and harmful and condemns it utterly. I make the plea that every stress above the minimum required in any given labor should now be regarded as an unnecessary and unjustified risk to the tissues and therefore should also be vigorously condemned.

SUMMARY

A suggestion is put forward that a review of the present management of the normal second stage of labor is timely and that reform is required.

Some detailed observations are made concerning the completely spontaneous second stage. Particular attention is drawn to an interval which occurs after the onset of each contraction before the natural impulse to strain begins.

The results of a pilot clinical survey are given in which only a minority (11 per cent) of patients showed any need for teaching or coercion in pushing.

The survey showed that the idea is wrong that labor must be unduly prolonged if instruction in pushing is not given.

A regime which reserved instruction for those cases who proved their need for it, showed a considerable reduction in the incidence of both forceps delivery and perineal laceration.

Theoretical reasons are also put forward which suggest that too early and too hard pushing even in the second stage may be harmful to the maternal tissues.

A plea is made for a more vigorous policy to eliminate hurry and unnecessary straining from the conduct of the normal second stage of labor.

I wish to record my thanks to Sister Harry and Sister Bolton of the Sussex Maternity Hospital for their loyal cooperation and untiring help in collecting these figures for me, and to all the doctors and midwives who have cooperated with me there and elsewhere in trying to prove the value of this procedure.

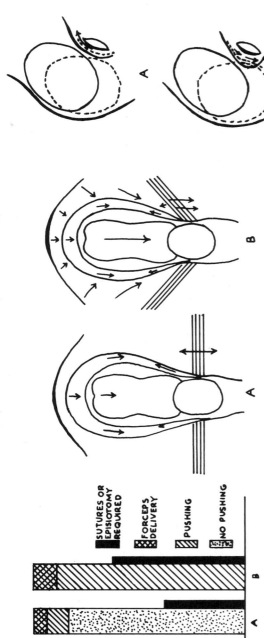

FIG. 1
Results of Labor

A. No suggestion of pushing
allowed unless it was proved
to be necessary.

B. Pushing encouraged in the
usual way.

FIG. 2
Stress on transverse
cervical ligaments.

A. Uterine force acting alone.

B. Secondary powers used
while presenting part still
gripped by cervix or vagina.

FIG. 3
Stress on anterior
vaginal wall.

A. Straining late in the
contraction only.

B. Straining from the onset
of the contraction.

-31-

REFERENCES

Browne, FJ (1955): Antenatal and Postnatal Care 8th edition. Churchill, London. p. 447.

Claye, AM (1955) in Holland E (ed.): British Obstetric and Gynaecological Practice Vol. I. Heinemann, London. p. 141.

Danforth DM (1947): Am J Obstet Gynecol 53:541.

Danforth DM and Ivy AC (1949): Am J Obstet Gynecol 57:839.

De Soldenhoff R (1956): Practitioner 176:413.

Greenhill JP (1955): Obstetrics 11th edition. Saunders, Philadelphia. pp. 184-186.

Jeffcoate TNA (1950): Brit Med J 1:1361.

Kanton HJ, Miller JE and Dunlap JC (1949): Am J Obstet Gynecol 58:354.

Malpas P (1955): Genital Prolapse and Allied Conditions. Harvey & Blythe, London. p. 42.

Malpas P, Jeffcoate TNA and Lister W (1949): J Obstet Gynaecol Br Emp 56:949.

Miles M (1956): Textbook for Midwives 2nd edition. Livingstone, Edinburgh. pp. 294-295.

Moir JC (ed.) (1956): Munro Kerr's Operative Obstetrics 6th edition. Balliere, Tindall & Cox, London. pp. 109 and 913.

Watson BP (1924): Br Med J 2:566.

3. Pelvic Floor Awareness.

Sheila Kitzinger, M.Litt.

Pelvic floor awareness is more than good muscle tone; it is the ability to gain and give pleasure in lovemaking and intercourse; to spontaneously open up to release the baby during birth; and to restore function and tone after birth. Here, a British childbirth educator and anthropologist explains what women need to know about their pelvic floors and specifically how they can be helped to learn.

Despite its name, the pelvic floor musculature is not really at all like a floor. The muscles are attached to the cradle of bone which forms the pelvis at the level of the outlet rather like a sail attached to a mast. And, like a sail, their direction can be changed.

This mobility of the pelvic floor, its responsiveness and active functioning, is essential for good tone. When muscles are not used they invariably slacken and become weak. Because human beings are upright, rather than on all fours, pelvic floor tone is necessary in order to support all the pelvic contents -- for a woman not only the bladder and rectum, but the uterus too, and, at one remove, the abdominal organs. (Four-legged mammals support these organs with the muscles of the abdominal wall.)

There are three openings through these bands of muscle fibers--the anus, the vagina and the urethra. The muscles circle round them roughly in the shape of a figure 8. [See Figure 1 in "The Midline Episiotomy" by Y. Gordon in this volume.] Any forceful, uncoordinated pushing subjects these muscle bands to strain. In much the same way, a racking cough puts stress on the pelvic floor, too.

When anything is released from the body through these orifices, the muscles need to be relaxed. If they do not relax function is inhibited, the process of letting the object pass through is delayed and pain is experienced.

Pelvic floor awareness enables a woman first to increase muscle tone so that she has what can be thought of as "good internal posture" and to release the muscles so that there is smooth, coordinated activity and she can open herself at will. Exercises for the pelvic floor are sometimes taught exclusively during pregnancy in order to strengthen and tone and to achieve rehabilitation after childbirth, to the neglect of this other, "giving" function of the pelvic floor. Moreover, with the present popular emphasis on exercises during pregnancy and the number of books published which stress the need for firm muscles as a prerequisite to easy childbirth, many women assume that tight muscles are the goal. This is sometimes reinforced by

anxiety that their bodies may become slack and limp after
childbirth and that they will not recover their figures.
There may then be an obsessive concern to exercise and tone
the pelvic floor which can make harmonious psycho-physical
coordination in the second stage very difficult to achieve.
In childbirth education the focus should be on pelvic floor
activity rather than merely on either contraction or
relaxation of the musculature. Just as the muscles of our
faces move, in an interplay of contraction and release
resulting in different expressions, the muscles of the
pelvic floor can be active in the same way. The pelvic floor
can come alive. It can be a vital, expressive part of a
woman's body. This is quite different from just "doing
exercises."

In the early days of childbirth education, teaching
about the pelvic floor rarely included discussion of its
function in lovemaking and intercourse. Women were taught
simply that these muscles were used to stop the stream of
urine and that they could test their strength when on the
toilet. Though this emphasized the function of the muscles
in terms of retention and evacuation of body contents, in
the context of childbirth it directed attention to the
expulsion of the fetus almost as if it, too, were waste
matter that had to be got out of the body. Today attitudes
have changed and probably most teachers refer to the use of
the pelvic muscles in sexual intercourse. Even so, muscle
contractions are sometimes described as if they were
employed solely to give pleasure to a male partner. The
sensory pleasure a woman gains from stimulation of nerve
ends in these muscles may be neglected. Together with
clitoral stimulation, pelvic floor movements can, for some
pre-orgasmic women, open the way to the experience of
orgasm. This occurs because strong activity in the pelvic
floor tends to stimulate the spongy pads of tissue between
the anterior vaginal wall and the urethra and the perineal
tissue between the posterior vaginal wall and the anus. (The
former is the location of the so-called G-spot, the latter
the area which is excited during anal stimulation.)

LEAVE IT TO INSTINCT?

Recently there has been a swing away from emphasis on
detailed instruction and a much greater stress on emotional
and experiential aspects of childbirth. This is all to the
good. It is sometimes asserted, however, that all
preparation for birth detracts from the reality of lived
experience and that to teach anything is to interfere with
spontaneous, natural behavior in labor.

Yet all activity in childbirth, both on the part of the
woman in labor and that of her attendants, is shaped by
culture. None of it is purely "natural" in the sense that

other animal behavior is natural. And it is doubtful whether any woman enters labor with a mind completely blank of all ideas about it. Though it is undoubtedly true that a woman who is able to act spontaneously, who can get in any position she wants, who feels safe and among friends and is not afraid of the intense sensations she is experiencing can usually release and open up for her baby to be born, most women do not give birth under these conditions. In an alien and institutional environment, with strangers coming in and out, often forced to adopt an uncomfortable and unphysiological position for delivery, they resist sensations in the perineum as the baby's head descends and do not feel free to behave spontaneously. Many are afraid of dirtying the bed. Many fear that they will split. There may also be after-effects from a previous birth experience which resulted in emotional or physical trauma. It must be taken into account, too, that routine practices involved in management, including limitations on time in the second stage, commands to push and "try harder" and concern to avoid a tear at all costs, together often impose on the laboring woman a strictly defined culture of childbirth which limits her freedom to do as she wishes, controls her actions and may also introduce other peoples' anxieties.

It follows that it is not enough for women to approach childbirth confident and free from fear. They also need to be able to cope with a social situation in which it may be difficult for them to be assertive or to act with any spontaneity.

Michel Odent has shown that a loving and emotionally supportive environment for birth and an upright position during the second stage together almost eliminate the need for episiotomy. If a woman does have a tear under such conditions it is usually just a small nick in the surface skin (a first degree laceration), frequently involving the labia rather than perineal tissue. He believes that when women can revert to what he calls "the primitive brain" in labor, childbirth education is irrelevant. (Michel Odent, Genese de l'homme ecologique Epi, 1979.)

Yet some women find it impossible to do this, even in a loving environment, because they are not able to trust their bodies. One important element in having the confidence to do this in labor is positive pelvic floor awareness. Pregnancy need not be just a waiting time. It provides an opportunity for a woman to explore and find her own body rhythms and get in touch with her feelings.

UNDERSTANDING THE PELVIC FLOOR

Pelvic floor muscles are spontaneously active when the bowels and bladder are emptied. A woman does not need to know where they are or how they work in order to use them effectively. Yet even in these functions anxiety, fear and undue haste can inhibit spontaneous activity and interfere with the rhythmic nature of contraction and release of the muscles. Normal pleasurable activity is also lost with constipation, cystitis, vaginal infections such as thrush, if there is a cystocele or a rectocele and, above all, following perineal injuries. Painful intercourse and sexual assault may also result in overpowering anxiety which makes it difficult to use the pelvic floor muscles voluntarily and with ease. They may be held clamped tight and "frozen".

During intense sexual arousal the pelvic floor contracts and relaxes in an accelerating rhythm and immediately preceding orgasm these contractions become staccato, each alternating with a few seconds' release. In multiple orgasm the pelvic floor is tightly clasped as the woman reaches the climax of each wave of excitement, released after she is over the crest of the wave and this is followed by further staccato contractions accompanying the next wave of desire.

It cannot be taken for granted, however, that experiencing orgasm enables a woman to be fully aware of these muscles. For some women orgasm appears to be a vague generalized feeling, without specific or powerful genital sensation. (Sheila Kitzinger, Woman's Experience of Sex Putnam, 1983.) Others experience a localized climax but do not particularly value isolated genital sensations. They are emotionally distanced from it, and prefer more general arousal and release. There is no one "right" way to have an orgasm.

Some women find it difficult to use pelvic floor muscles voluntarily during lovemaking because a male partner ejaculates too quickly and they either are reluctant to move at all lest the activity over-excite the man or, because he does not continue love-making after ejaculation, do not get a chance to let the muscles "play" following his orgasm. Any pelvic muscle activity can become threatening to a woman who feels she should be passive or hold herself rigid for her partner's sake in order to prolong intercourse or because, for religious or cultural reasons, it is wrong.

So there are many reasons why pelvic floor awareness and coordination in childbirth bring stress and challenge and cannot always be left to instinct. Though the childbirth educator will often not know what the implications of pelvic muscle activity are for each woman, it is important that she recognize the possible effects of the way in which she talks about the pelvic floor and the kind of exercises she teaches for it.

SOME WAYS TO TALK ABOUT
AND EXPLORE THESE MUSCLES

Bands of muscle fibers, strong and flexible like elastic, circle round the opening from the bladder, the vagina and the anus. The anus, particularly, has a strong sphincter which can close it entirely. "It's quite easy for us to 'wink' with our anuses." The vagina does not have a sphincter like this. Muscle fibers encircle the vagina further up inside. It feels as if there is a muscle ring about half-way up and it is when this ring is tightened that a woman can make a "kiss inside" and can grip her lover's penis or finger during lovemaking.

It is important that the childbirth educator teaching couples together does not discuss the pelvic floor in such a way that the men feel that they are merely observers. With all other birth education teachers are becoming increasingly concerned to help men understand as much of the woman's experience as possible. And they, too, can explore pelvic floor movements. The bands of muscle fiber which are equivalent to those about half-way up inside the vagina coil round the root of the penis, so that when they are contracted it lifts slightly toward the pubic bone.

Because the muscles form a figure 8 it is impossible to isolate contractions "at the front" from those "at the back". A strong contraction tightens both circles of muscle so that they change from being round to being almond-shaped. Simultaneously the "cross-band of fibers", the transverse perineal muscle, is drawn up and forward toward the pubic bone, rather as when an old-fashioned roll-top desk is opened.

Unlike a real floor, the pelvic floor has different layers of muscle higher inside. It is these which perform the main work of supporting the bladder and uterus. They are slanted at different angles to each other rather like stage scenery. So as they are tightened pressure can be noted at varying points in the pelvis.

THE ELEVATOR EXERCISE

"A simple way of helping recognition of these deeper strata of muscle is to imagine that you have 'an elevator inside' which can start at the ground floor and go up to, say, five floors. Let the elevator ascend floor by floor. Wait at each floor and notice how it feels. Begin from the first floor and go up to the second. Can you feel the pressure? Now from the second to the third. (Go on breathing though!) From the third to the fourth. Notice the pressure against your bladder. You will feel this especially if your bladder is rather full. Now the fourth to the fifth (but don't try to pull your pelvic muscles up with your shoulders!) And now down...from the fifth to the fourth, the fourth to the third, the third to the second -- and to the ground floor.

"The elevator can go down to the basement, too. Now press the muscles down. Notice how that feels. This is exactly the movement you make in labor as you push the baby out.

"Then come up to the second floor again so that you always finish with good muscle tone, never with a flop and a sag."

The childbirth educator can also use this exercise as a basis for discussion about physical sensation in the second stage of labor and the mechanics of pushing. It is sometimes thought, and indeed taught, by many birth attendants, that in order to push effectively a woman must contract her abdominal muscles and suck them in toward her spine. This is not, however, what she does spontaneously in the expulsive stage of labor. With spontaneous pushing only the lateral abdominals are contracted, and that contraction is static and occurs only at the height of the urge to push. The pelvic floor muscles bulge downward and the perineum is pressed out, rather like a bag heavy with dripping jelly or cream cheese or like a sponge saturated with water. A pregnant woman whose breasts are heavy can sometimes get this feeling if she cups a hand underneath the breast at the same time that she releases the pelvic floor and allows it to press down.

When the pelvic floor descends a woman opens up to let the baby be born and her lower abdomen bulges out quite spontaneously. She does not have to push it out. The teacher can suggest that women place one hand firmly just above the pubic symphysis, over the base of the abdomen, and note what they feel is happening as they do the elevator movement with the pelvic floor. "What do you feel as the elevator goes up? . . . . Yes, it is sucked in . . . . Now try going down to the ground floor...and now further still to the basement. What has happened? . . . . Yes, there is pressure under your hand because you are bulging out there."

This action can also be observed by the support person attending the class with the woman if he or she rests a hand over her pubis and lower abdomen and she does the elevator movement while the hand is held in this position.

If a woman has an epidural this is a way in which she can be helped to push in a coordinated manner in the absence of any spontaneous urge to do so. Once the presenting part is on the perineum -- and to do so before wastes energy -- her labor companion, nurse or midwife places a hand over the lower abdomen and she presses it outward several times at the height of each contraction.

This action of the descent of the pelvic floor and expansion of the lower abdomen allows perineal tissues to fan out progressively, like a knife-pleated skirt swinging wide or a fan spreading open. The presenting part, usually the fetal occiput, presses through like a ball, exerting equal pressure all round and easing open these tissues wider and wider. A woman can become aware of this pressure on the perineum if she rests a hand firmly over it as she allows the pelvic floor to descend.

She will feel even more pressure if she tries the same movement as she crouches or squats. In the second stage of labor a woman spontaneously seeks a position which is comfortable, and this is usually an upright or semi-upright posture in which she has gravity to help her. If contractions are very powerful and are coming fast, however, she sometimes prefers to be on all fours, to lie curved on her side, or to recline with her head and shoulders well raised.

When a woman is deliberately pushing because she is commanded or coaxed to do so, or because she has learned previously that she must, great stress may be put on the pelvic floor and perineal tissues. This is especially the case if she bears down for a prolonged period, holding her breath at the same time. The result is that the perineal tissues become pale and shiny. The whole area is numb since the pressure is so great that both blood supply and nerve impulses are cut off. The perineum looks as if it were a balloon being blown up and becoming more and more shiny before it pops. It is under these circumstances that it is helpful for an attendant to employ a technique of "guarding" the perineum with hand pressure or ironing it out with an oiled finger. If pushing is never mentioned, however, and a woman only pushes when she must -- and then only for as long as she must -- perineal trauma is reduced or eliminated and techniques of supporting the perineum, and of easing the baby's head over the perineum, are often unnecessary. The emphasis is on opening up, not on pushing.

Pelvic floor muscles can also be discussed in relation to muscles around the mouth. The mouth can be held tight or released and the muscles used in a variety of different expressions. As women did the elevator exercise they may have been aware that as they tightened the pelvic floor muscles those around the mouth also tended to tighten. As they released the pelvic floor, these muscles also relaxed. There is an association between the mouth and the vagina. This is why deliberately releasing the mouth and jaw as the head approaches the perineum can help pelvic release, too. When a woman shouts or cries out the same thing happens. Thus letting sound out can help pelvic relaxation. Conversely, holding sound back because a woman wants to be on her best behavior or because noise is considered shameful can actually prevent her letting go.

The teacher can also extend the mouth-vagina association and describe pelvic floor activity in terms of "expressions". Muscles of the face move as part of ordinary living and our interaction with other people. The pelvic floor muscles can be mobile in much the same way. When a woman is severely depressed her pelvic floor invariably sags, along with the muscles of her face. Good muscle tone is like a pelvic floor smile. A useful reminder may be to "greet each morning with a pelvic foor smile."

An exercise which focuses on varied movement in the pelvic floor I have given the name Happy Birthday. "Imagine that you want to write "Happy Birthday" using your pelvic floor muscles. When you are at the top of a letter your muscles are contracted tightest. When you descend to the bottom of a letter they are bulged down. Please try to write clearly!"

The teacher slowly says the letters one by one. She will notice some people moving their mouths, tongues or jaws to help control movement in the pelvic floor and can draw attention to this as obvious when attempts are made to shape letters like the "o"s of the double p. There is usually laughter when she encourages them to "dot the i."

Pelvic floor muscles also tend to work in association with muscles of the inner thighs -- the adductors -- and with those of the buttocks -- the glutei. "Press your knees and the tops of your legs firmly together and at the same time pull in your pelvic floor muscles as high as they will go. Now see if you can relax your legs while keeping your pelvic floor muscles tight . . . . It is difficult because the inner thigh muscles and pelvic muscles tend to work together. It is important to remember this when in labor. When your inner thigh muscles are well relaxed it is much easier to relax the pelvic floor . . . . Now press your buttocks tightly together as if you had a sheet of writing paper between them and somebody was trying to take it away from you! At the same time pull in the muscles of the pelvic floor as high as they will go. Now try to release your buttocks while at the same time keeping your pelvic floor muscles tight . . . . You will see that this is very difficult, too. It is because the buttock muscles and the pelvic floor muscles also tend to work in association with each other. So in labor it is important to keep your buttock muscles relaxed. The pelvic floor muscles are then much more likely to be relaxed too."

Checking pelvic floor tone is usually suggested in terms of interrupting a stream of urine. I have already said that this emphasizes the retentive function of the pelvic floor to the exclusion of its opening function. It may be better, therefore, to suggest that a woman choose a time when she is quiet and relaxed to slip a finger inside (oiled if she prefers) so that she can herself feel her pelvic muscles squeezing and can also press down on her finger as if to push it out. She can explore the same muscular activity using a sexual partner's finger or penis.

ACTIVATING THE PELVIC FLOOR AFTER CHILDBIRTH

There is no evidence that doing strenuous pelvic floor exercises in the days immediately following delivery improves pelvic tone. Rather the opposite. Women who exercise in the first weeks, according to one study, have less good tone when tested after delivery. (Lewis Mehl et al., Episiotomy: Facts, Fictions, Figures and Alternatives, Compulsory Hospitalization: Freedom of Choice in Childbirth NAPSAC, 1979.)
There may be advantages, however, in making exploratory movements so that a woman feels in touch with this part of her body and that it is in good working order. The sense of being in control of one's body, able to feel and activate it, can be important psychologically because awareness of this part of the body is integral to a more general sense of physical well-being. After she has had a baby a woman often feels that her whole pelvic region has become a medical object and the property of doctors and nurses. It is an image of sickness and of diseased or mutilated organs. When there has been perineal trauma or surgery this sense of alienation from her genital area may be so powerful that she does not want to look at or touch her perineum or vagina and is frightened of what she might find. (Sheila Kitzinger, Woman's Experience of Sex Putnam, 1983.)
It often takes some weeks before a woman can fully mobilize her pelvic muscles, especially after suturing of the perineum, and exercising may cause pain. This pain often persists for three months or longer after delivery if she has been stitched too tightly, not allowing for the swelling which follows injury to the perineum. Exploratory movements should never be done beyond the point of pain.
A respiratory tract infection with a cough, or straining on the toilet, delays rehabilitation of the pelvic floor. The idea of releasing the muscles, rather than pushing feces out, can be helpful in coping with initial constipation.
When her pelvic floor lacks tone a woman may feel that there is something heavy hanging down and be unable to contract her muscles at all, or she may be able to contract slightly but the muscles tremble if she attempts a sustained contraction. The teacher can suggest that she may find it easier to explore activity when she is not upright, so that the weight of her own pelvic contents is not pressing on the sling of muscles. She may be more comfortable lying down or lying on her back with her knees bent and lower legs raised onto a chair so that her pelvis is tilted and her feet are

above the level of her pelvis. It is often possible to feel movement in this position when it cannot be felt sitting or standing. If a muscle trembles it is an indication that it should be released. There should be a gradual progression to stronger and longer contractions and each woman should be guided by her own body. The teacher's task is to help her get more sensitively in touch and confident in her body, not to institute a gymnastic drill. She can point out that when a muscle is bruised, blood loaded with carbon dioxide lies in the "pockets" in the muscle, rather like water in a sponge: "If, as you lie in the bathtub, you have a soapy sponge, the more you squeeze the sponge under water, the more the soap goes out and fresh water comes in. In much the same way, rhythmic movements in pelvic floor muscles help them to get rid of blood which is loaded with waste products so that fresh, oxygenated blood can flow in. And this new blood helps the muscle to heal."

4. Influence of Maternal Bearing-Down Efforts During Second Stage on Fetal Well-Being.

Roberto Caldeyro-Barcia, M.D.

(This paper was first published in Kaleidoscope of Childbearing: Preparation, Birth and Nurturing, in 1978 by Pennypress, Inc., and is reprinted here with the author's permission.)

Prolonged breathholding and straining by the mother are expected and encouraged by most birth attendants, who assume such efforts will result in a more rapid delivery, and thus benefit the fetus. But what of the decreased oxygen supply available if the mother seldom takes a breath? What are the effects of straining? Here a well known researcher in the physiology of childbirth describes potentially harmful effects to the fetus from such bearing-down efforts.

Recently the question was raised of the effects on the fetus of strong and prolonged bearing-down efforts combined with breath-holding. Our preliminary investigations indicate that prolonged bearing-down efforts by the mother during the second stage of labor seem to be dangerous for the fetus. By "prolonged," I mean lasting more than 6 or 7 seconds. Closure of the glottis causes an increase in intrathoracic pressure which is also dangerous.

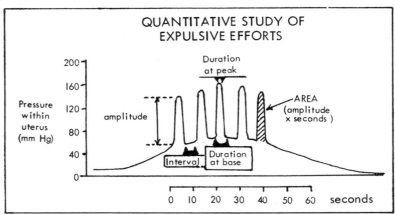

FIGURE I. In this diagram we can see the intrauterine pressure measured in mm Hg and time measured in seconds. The pressure of the uterine contraction increases to almost 80 mm Hg and gradually decreases. Each of five bearing-down efforts of the mother adds 70 to 80 mm Hg of intrauterine pressure to the contraction pressure.

The duration of bearing-down efforts (as indicated in Figure 1 by the sharp rise in intrauterine pressure) was measured and the best results, in terms of fetal well-being, were obtained when this duration was between 4 and 6 seconds. The amplitude (or rise in intrauterine pressure) which women produced spontaneously was between 70 and 80 mm Hg above the pressure already built by the uterine contraction. The increased pressure during the bearing-down efforts results from the contraction of the muscles of the abdominal wall. They cause a rapid rise in intrauterine pressure, while the contraction of the uterus is a slow and gradual increase and decrease in intrauterine pressure.

Following are a few records (Figures 2, 3, 4 and 5) showing contractions and the bearing-down efforts related to fetal heart rate.

It is very important to note that all commercial monitors now available record pressures only to 100 mm Hg (as seen in line B of Figures 2 and 3). The amplitude of the bearing-down efforts cannot be recorded. When they go above 100 mm Hg, nothing is being recorded except the horizontal lines at the top of each bearing-down effort, indicating 100 mm Hg or more. Partly because of this limitation in the technology, bearing-down efforts and their effects have never been studied by anyone. This is why we changed to more sensitive instruments which can record up to 200 mm Hg of intrauterine pressure (see line C in Figures 2 and 3).

Bearing-down efforts play a very important role in the outcome of labor and the welfare of the fetus. Referring to Figure 2 once more, the first bearing-down effort is longer than those following. We had asked the mother to make a prolonged bearing-down effort. It lasted about 9 seconds whereas those following, which she did spontaneously, lasted 5 to 6 seconds. This makes a big difference to the fetus. When the duration of the bearing-down effort is longer than 15 seconds (much longer than the longest one seen here), the hypoxic effects on the fetus are much more marked than we see here. In this case we can see that each bearing-down effort caused a corresponding fall in fetal heart rate. These are Type 1 Dips (early decelerations) caused by the fetal head being compressed more strongly while the woman was bearing down. The fetal heart rate then recovered after the last bearing-down effort was performed. The last four bearing-down efforts which were spontaneously and normally performed by the mother had no damaging hypoxic effects on the fetus. The first, longer one caused a longer lasting fall in fetal heart rate. This can be damaging as we shall see in a moment.

Figure 3 shows another contraction in the same labor as Figure 2. All the woman's bearing-down efforts were spontaneous and effects on the fetal heart rate were

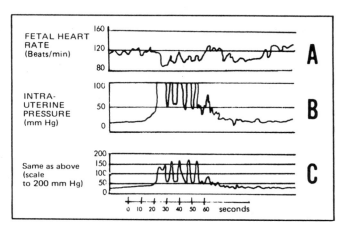

FIGURE 2. In this figure we see a record of a contraction; B shows intrauterine pressure on a scale from 0 to 100 mm Hg; C shows the same thing on a more amplified scale of from 0 to 200 mm Hg. This lower scale, with its increased sensitivity of the recording enables us to measure the uterine contraction plus the entire amplitude of each bearing-down effort. The peaks of the bearing-down efforts go up to about 165 mm Hg. The peak of the contraction reaches about 65 mm Hg.

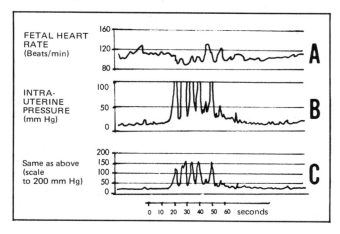

FIGURE 3. In this figure, we see a similar record of a later contraction in the same labor as the previous figure. All bearing-down efforts here were spontaneous, lasting about 5 seconds. There is only a transient effect on the fetal heart rate during each bearing-down effort, but no fall in fetal heart rate after the contraction (late decelerations), which are the dangerous ones.

transient and did not last beyond the contraction. Decelerations that persist after the contraction's end are considered to be the dangerous ones.

Figure 4 shows a contraction from another labor, with the maternal femoral artery pressure (systolic and diastolic) and the fetal heart rate.

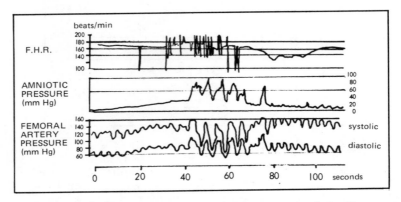

FIGURE 4. Here we come to a very important point. Here we have a recording of a contraction (the middle record), with 6 bearing-down efforts, the fetal heart rate (above) and the maternal femoral artery pressure (below). The upper line records systolic pressure; the lower line records diastolic pressure. At the beginning of each bearing-down effort there is a short-lasting rise in both systolic and diastolic blood pressure. Then, as the bearing-down effort continues, there is a marked drop in both systolic and diastolic blood pressure, which recurs with each bearing-down effort.

At the beginning of each bearing-down effort there is a short-lasting rise in both systolic and diastolic blood pressure. The mechanism involved here is as follows: a bearing-down effort involves breathholding and closing of the glottis resulting in increased intrathoracic pressure (clearly seen as congestion in the face of the mother.)

The increased intrathoracic pressure produces a drop in venous return to the heart, a drop in cardiac output, a drop in maternal arterial pressure (to about 70 mm Hg systolic and less than 50 mm Hg diastolic). The longer the bearing-down effort, the more marked the fall in arterial pressure of the mother. The fall in arterial pressure causes a drop in perfusion of blood in the placenta and a drop in oxygen getting to the fetus -- fetal hypoxia.

In Figure 5, some of the bearing-down efforts were very long, and caused fetal hypoxia as demonstrated on the recording of fetal heart rate as a late deceleration (occurring after the contraction) and recovering slowly.

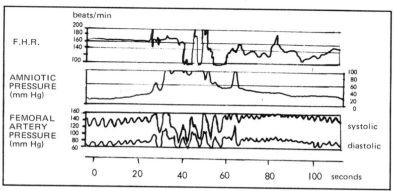

FIGURE 5. We see a similar recording to Figure 4, showing even longer and stronger bearing-down efforts. They were so strong they went beyond the limits of the recording system (100 mm Hg). The effort lasted for about 18 seconds, during which the intrauterine pressure never went down to normal. The arterial pressure dropped to around 70/50 mm Hg. This greatly reduced blood flow to the placenta and produced marked fetal hypoxia as reflected in the fetal heart rate tracing. After the end of the contraction there was a fall in fetal heart rate to between 100 and 130 beats per minute (before the contraction it had been at about 160 beats per minute) which lasted long after the contraction. This is considered a prolonged late deceleration and produced fetal acidosis.

Ironically, it is this fetal hypoxia and acidosis seen in the second stage of labor that is given as the reason why second stage should be very short. It is recognized as being dangerous to the fetus, but it has not been understood until now that our instructions to the mother in second stage to bear down long and hard are causing this fetal hypoxia and acidosis! Her spontaneous efforts usually are within physiological limits — about 5 or 6 seconds long.

Not only is there a drop in maternal arterial pressure, but because the mother is holding her breath (closing the glottis), the drop in blood pressure is accompanied by a fall in the oxygen content of her arterial blood. The result, then, of prolonged bearing-down effort with breath-holding is not only reduced blood flow to the placenta, but also decreased oxygen content in the blood that does reach the placenta. It is the combination of these two factors which produce fetal hypoxia.

Fetal hypoxia can be avoided if the mother bears down physiologically as she feels the need, and without closing her glottis or prolonging the bearing-down. We have found consistently that both fetus and neonate are in much better shape, both clinically and biochemically. At birth we measure samples of umbilical arterial blood for pH and pO_2. The neonate is much more likely to be acidotic and to have a low oxygen content when the mother has been bearing down for too long, with great strength and with the glottis closed.

This is another way we have been interfering with the normal second stage of labor. These studies are not yet finished, but we have learned that we should recommend that parturient women be instructed to bear down as they feel the need, without trying to produce very strong or prolonged (longer than 6 seconds) efforts, and without complete closure of the glottis.

Second stage proceeds more slowly when the woman bears down in this way, but the fetus is in excellent condition. I do not see any reason for speeding up second stage, when the fetus is handling it well. Another advantage to a longer second stage is that it gives the perineum more time to stretch slowly and the need for episiotomy is very markedly reduced.

5. Maternal Positions for Second Stage.

Katherine C. Carr, R.N., C.N.M., M.S.

In North America, the positions usually adopted by laboring women are supine or semi-sitting with the knees drawn up toward the shoulders, either held by the woman, support people, or stirrups. These are not positions chosen by the woman, but by her birth attendants. They are frequently uncomfortable, inefficient, and may cause fetal hypoxia. Here, an American Nurse-Midwife discusses a variety of possible maternal positions with their implications for management.

Women throughout history and throughout the world have used a variety of positions for giving birth. The following is a discussion and review of some of the most commonly used birthing positions, the advantages and disadvantages of each, indications for use and instructions for the woman and her care provider. There is no single perfect or correct position. Each position has positive and negative points. Each should be utilized to facilitate the birth of the infant in a safe and comfortable manner.

The upright positions (standing, supported or suspended squat and leaning forward or crouching) with the trunk in a vertical plane, have been the rule for many cultures.[1-3] The advantages of the upright positions are numerous. The most obvious advantage is the aid of gravity. According to Newton's Law of Gravity, it is easier for an object to fall toward the earth's surface than to slide parallel to it. A mechanical advantage exists when the fetus is expelled downward, rather than along a horizontal plane.[4] Supine hypotension syndrome due to vena caval compression by the pregnant uterus as well as aortal compression with its resulting maternal hypotension, are avoided in the upright positions. Thus uterine blood flow and fetal oxygenation are not reduced by the upright positions as they are by supine positions.[5,6] The upright positions also direct pressure on the fetal cranium toward the occipital fontanelle area (in an occiput anterior position). Embryonically, this is the oldest and best developed area of the fetal skull, and may be more capable of withstanding the stress of birth.[2]

Perhaps the most important advantage of the upright positions is the increased pelvic "mouldability" or movement of the pelvic architecture to maximize pelvic capacity. Radiographic studies have shown an increase in pelvic diameters in the squatting position.[7] Over one hundred years ago it was known that pelvic diameters in pregnant women vary with maternal position.[8] It has been shown that positions where the thighs are abducted and flexed at the hip joints cause the lower sacrum to swing backward, enlarging the sagittal diameter of the outlet. These positions also cause sliding movements of the sacroiliac joints, enlarging the transverse diameters of the pelvis at the midpelvis (spines) and outlet. The subpubic angle is also widened. Russell identifies the critical points to consider in maximizing these effects to enlarge pelvic capacity. The factors that must be present to increase "pelvic moulding" include abducted femora that act as levers to open the sacroiliac joints and the pelvic tilt position to cause backward movement of the sacrum.[9,10] This additional space in the pelvis due to a positional change facilitates internal rotation and descent.

The squatting position exerts maximum leverage for enlarging the pelvic diameters due to the increased weight on the femora. The half-squat, leaning forward or crouching and standing (with thighs abducted and legs slightly flexed) facilitate these same pelvic changes but to varying degrees. Such upright positions also allow a woman the freedom to shift her weight from side to side, to kneel on one knee or the other, and to adopt any number of asymmetrical positions. Such asymmetrical postures, adopted quite spontaneously by women, facilitate rotation and descent of the fetus.

In addition to enlarging pelvic diameters, maternal comfort may be enhanced by the upright positions, especially when backache is severe.

The upright positions also aid in the relaxation of the perineal musculature, which facilitates delivery over an intact perineum.

The disadvantages to the upright positions are few. Access to the perineum may be limited, as it is close to the floor with squatting and may be difficult to see. Raising the squatting area on a platform or having the woman squat in bed may help to solve this problem. Women will need to practice these positions prenatally and may need support to avoid toppling over. Of course, these positions are most useful in the unanesthetized woman, although they are sometimes possible in women who have a light epidural block. Occasionally, second stage can be quite rapid in the upright positions, leading to rapid expulsion of the fetus and perineal lacerations. In women with a history of precipitous second stage, upright positions are best avoided.

Upright positions may be indicated for primagravidae or when lack of progress is evident in second stage for more than 15-20 minutes. Other indications include the presence of a large fetus, small pelvis or malposition (especially OP or transverse arrest). Maternal comfort may be enhanced by a change of positions at any time. The upright positions facilitate the use of many comfort measures especially when back massage is needed.

Instructions for standing include knees slightly bent with feet apart for balance. Support on each side of the mother may be helpful, or she may wish to lean forward slightly with her arms around another person. It is easiest for the attendant to assist the birth from behind.

The supported squat or suspended squat requires an assistant or a support such as a birthing stool or a solid wall to lean against. The attendants may support the woman from behind, holding her under her arms, or the woman may brace herself against a wall. The attendants may also support the woman from the front or she may sit on a birthing stool or block. In any case, she does not support all of her own weight. Her hips are slightly but not completely flexed, and her thighs are not pressing on the uterine wall. This supported position may provide more comfort for the woman unused to or too tired to squat, but in need of an upright position to facilitate delivery.

When largely supported by a partner, the woman bears less of her weight. This may provide a unique advantage not offered by any other position -- a reduction in the forces which restrict mobility of the pelvic joints. When side-lying, semi-sitting, standing or squatting, there are forces (pressure of body weight resting on a surface, or of muscular tension created by maintaining an unassisted position) which tend to "set" the pelvis, sometimes in an advantageous position, sometimes in a restrictive position. When supported from above in a semi-upright position, the woman is able to relax her lower body, reducing or eliminating any forces impinging on pelvic mobility, and possibly restricting beneficial movement. As the fetus descends, the skull can mold the pelvic joints as necessary.

The true squat requires that the thighs be flexed, abducted and against the sides of the uterus. The heels of the feet are flat on the floor and the woman is supporting her weight on the femora to facilitate the pelvic changes discussed above. It may be helpful to have a bar or pole available for the woman to hold onto to keep her balance. [See Appendix B for details on teaching and mastering the squatting position.]

Most women in the Western world must be prepared prenatally to assume various upright positions for giving birth. That preparation should continue during labor by encouraging ambulation and frequent position change. The upright positions for second stage will then become a normal part of giving birth, once again.

The recumbent positions for delivery (lithotomy, side-lying and semi-sitting or propped), with the trunk in a horizontal plane, will be reviewed next. Lithotomy is the most prevalent delivery position in obstetrics today. Historically, this position was developed to allow easy access for procedures such as forceps and vacuum extractor, episiotomy, fetal monitoring and use of analgesia and anesthesia. The increasing use of such procedures, coupled with the invention of the delivery table, made it more critical for the birth attendant to have quick and ready access to the perineum. Certainly, for obstetric operations the lithotomy position has the advantage of good visibility, access to the perineum and easier maintenance of asepsis. It can be comfortable and convenient for the attendant as well. However, the lithotomy position has been criticized for many reasons. Its relationship with supine hypotension syndrome and aortal compression with resulting fetal effects are well documented.[3,6,12]

The lithotomy position has also been linked to increased perineal lacerations.[13] The over-enthusiastic raising and abducting of the legs or placing the thighs on the abdomen (in a supine position) does not increase the pelvic diameters but rather decreases them by pushing the sacrum forward. The skin and fascia of the perineum are attached to the flexion creases of the thighs. Such hyperflexion also makes the tissue of the perineum taut especially near the introitus, predisposing this area to laceration. Maternal discomfort is yet another problem due to the hyperabduction of the legs, torsion of the ligaments and pressure on the coccyx. Women very often complain of low back pain during and after use of the lithotomy position. Some women find this position embarrassing. This may inhibit their ability to relax the perineum for fear of expelling stool or urine. In short, it is not a natural position for women to assume.

Nevertheless, lithotomy is indicated for operative deliveries, necessary obstetrical procedures and difficult repairs.

Instructions for use of the lithotomy position should include the use of a wedge under the right hip, displacing the uterus to the left, to alleviate the supine hypotensive effects. The woman's feet should be dorsiflexed if cramping occurs in her calves. Discomfort of the legs, back and pelvis can be lessened by minimizing the length of time spent in lithotomy position.

None of the dorsal recumbent positions takes advantage of gravity to aid in the expulsion of the fetus. They also encourage the frontal lobes (in an occiput anterior position) on the brow of the fetus to present to the pelvis. As they are embryonically younger, they may be more apt to be damaged during the stress of birth.[2] Other recumbent positions including semi-sitting or propped (up to 30 degrees) and supine positioning have similar effects on the hemodynamics of mother and fetus to those of the lithotomy position (described above).

Side-lying or lateral recumbent (Sims position) avoids
the supine hypotensive effects of the other recumbent
positions. These positions have been long used in Britain.
The woman lies on her side, usually the left, and draws her
legs up against the uterus, or she allows the lower leg to
rest on the bed and draws up the right leg only or has it
supported by her partner or by a leg rest. The perineum is
very visible and accessible to the birth attendant in most
cases. It is an easy posture for the woman to assume as it
resembles a common sleep posture. It facilitates maternal
rest and comfort and does not give one the restricted
feeling of the lithotomy position. The perineal musculature
is more relaxed and the birth attendant can visualize the
presenting part quite well to help guide it over the
perineum.[14]

The side-lying position for delivery has been cited as
advantageous to mothers with congestive heart failure, hip
joint restriction and leg varicosities. It may be helpful
in slowing down those women with a rapid second stage. It is
also useful when the attendant has little or no assistance.
Women with extensive hemorrhoids may find this position the
most comfortable for pushing, as it allows for support of
the hemorrhoids with ice, heat or pressure.

The woman who is more comfortable lying down can be
helped to lie on her side and to draw up her knees if she
wishes. The bottom leg rests on the bed, while the upper leg
may be held by the woman, an assistant or placed on the
shoulder of the attendant. The woman can be encouraged to
watch the birth, as visibility by the woman is somewhat
better in the side-lying position than in supine positions.

Other positions for birthing that have been used are
the sitting, hands-and-knees and kneeling positions.
Although the trunk is in a vertical plane for sitting
(erect), there is little or no weightbearing by the legs to
provide the leverage needed to "mould" the pelvis and
enlarge the outlet. With kneeling, as long as the thighs are
abducted, "pelvic moulding" is caused by the femora acting
as levers, as with squatting. The forces of gravity are
helpful in these two positions as well. The hands-and-knees
position is more neutral in relation to gravitational
assistance. Supine hypotension syndrome can be avoided in
all three. The hands-and-knees position may be used when
severe backache or rectal pressure are present. It has also
been used effectively for breech delivery and relief of
shoulder dystocia.[15,16] It has been cited by obstetricians
as a helpful position in delivering obese patients.

Although there is no specific indication in the
literature for the use of the sitting position, other than
maternal preference or custom, some women may desire to use
this position. Instructions should include avoiding the
dorsal-recumbent (propped at less than 45 degrees) as this

may lead to supine hypotension or aortal compression. It may also be helpful to place arm supports at each side of the woman. If legs are crossed, this should be at the level of the ankles to encourage abduction of the thighs. Women often assume this position on the toilet for lack of birthing chairs.

In the hands-and-knees position the woman may rest on hands and knees, elbows and knees or chest and knees. The attendant must orient herself/himself to an upside-down delivery. This position provides the best visibility of the perineum.

With the kneeling position, support persons behind and in front of the woman are helpful. The woman may wish to lean back for a rest or be in need of massage or pressure from the attendants. The attendant assists with the birth from the front.

Using a variety of maternal positions for second stage may at times cause anxiety for the practitioner unfamiliar with delivery technique in positions other than lithotomy. One solution to this problem is to encourage the woman to take various positions until delivery is imminent, at which time she can assume the position of the practitioner's choice. It would be far more desirable for practitioners to develop the ability to manage births in a variety of positions.

During second stage, women should be encouraged to assume various postures to facilitate maternal comfort, ensure progress and most importantly, maintain fetal well-being. If at any time, there is lack of descent in second stage for 15-20 minutes, the woman should be encouraged to assume an upright position. Some types of fetal distress are remedied by positional changes as well. Extreme maternal discomfort may be alleviated by a position change and progress in second stage. Many obstetrical interventions can be avoided by following the examples of various birthing positions used by our foremothers.

REFERENCES

1. Engelmann, G. Labor among Primitive Peoples. St. Louis: JH Chambers & Company, 1882.

2. Position during labor & delivery: history and perspective. Liu Y. J Nurs Midwif 24:23-6, May-June 1979.

3. Alternative positions for childbirth--part II: the second stage of labor. Roberts J. J Nurs Midwif 25:13-19, Sept-Oct 1980.

4. The application of certain principles of physics to the physiology of delivery. Howard FH. West J Surg Obstet Gynecol 62:607-609, 1954.

5. Aortal compression by the uterus in late human pregnancy. Bieniarz J, et al. Am J Obstet Gynecol 100(2):203-217, Jan 1968.

6. Hansen J and Ueland K. "Maternal cardiovascular dynamics during pregnancy & parturition." In Parturition & Perinatology. F Marx (ed.). Philadelphia: FA Davis Co., 1973.

7. The mechanism of labour. Borrell U and Fernstrom I. Radio Clin N Am 5:73-85, 1967.

8. The behavior of the pelvic articulations in the mechanisms of parturition. Duncan JM. Dublin J Med Soc 18:60-69, 1854.

9. Moulding of the pelvic outlet. Russell JGB. J Obstet Gynaecol Br Commonw 76:817-820, 1969.

10. The rationale of primitive delivery positions. Russell JGB. Br J Obstet Gynaecol 89:712-715, 1982.

11. Employing Physiologic Principles to Manage Labor and Prevent Complications. Simkin P. Seattle: Pennypress, 1984.

12. Effect of labor on uterine blood flow. Gneiss FC. Am J Obstet Gynecol 93:917, 1965.

13. Factors associated with the occurence of perineal lacerations. Fischer S. J Nurs Midwif 24:1, Jan-Feb 1979.

14. Practical considerations for the routine application of left lateral Sims' position for vaginal delivery. Irwin H. Am J Obstet Gynecol 131:129-133, 1978.

15. Moir J. Munro Kerr's Operative Obstetrics, 7th Edition. Baltimore: The Williams & Wilkins Co., 1964.

16. "The Farm Midwives." Video presentation on Management of Shoulder Dystocia. The Farm: Summertown, Tennessee, 1981.

6. The Management of Labor: A Midwife's View.

Chloe Fisher, S.R.N., S.C.M., M.T.D.

DeLee compared the stress of delivery to that of falling on a woman's perineum and the effect of birth on the baby to that of having one's head crushed in a door. He asserted that "labor is pathogenic, disease producing, and anything pathogenic is pathologic or abnormal."[1]

In this chapter a nursing officer for community midwifery describes a different approach to the second stage.

How has it come about that such a high proportion of women receive episiotomies? During the last twenty years or so the percentage of women giving birth in hospitals with obstetricians in charge has risen enormously. Previously they had been the responsibility of midwives and general practitioners either at home or in small cottage hospital-type general practitioner units. During this time the permissible duration of the second stage for primigravida has become shorter and shorter -- even to as little as thirty minutes. A major reason for the increase in episiotomies, therefore has been the midwife's attempt to enable the woman in her care achieve a spontaneous delivery in the limited time allowed -- knowing that otherwise she must hand her delivery over to the obstetrician to be delivered by forceps. Simultaneously, there has been much discussion about the merits of episiotomies as a measure to prevent future pelvic floor problems -- though there has been no evidence to support this. We have now reached the stage where a small tear is considered evidence of poor delivery technique but to perform an episiotomy is absolutely acceptable.

The shortening of the second stage seems to have arisen because of the fear that this is a period of great stress for the fetus -- so that the sooner the baby is born, the better. There is however, evidence that directed, long bearing-down effort by the woman can itself be the cause of fetal distress.[2] So it is possible that by urging women to bear down, often out of phase with their own spontaneous expulsive urges, an iatrogenic fetal distress has arisen. It is known that women who have an effective epidural may do well in the second stage if they are not instructed to push until the presenting part is on the perineum. Why then is this practice considered unsafe for a normal labor? (Many skilled midwives overcome this problem by not counting the onset of the second stage until they can see the presenting part!)

In addition to the direct effect on the fetus, Beynon showed as long ago as 1957 that women who were not directed

to push had a much higher rate of spontaneous deliveries
than those who were chivied. Maybe we are now entering a
period where we can turn away from the concept of a short,
violent second stage and make our objective a gentle
untraumatic one.

Now that we are realizing that the pain caused by an
episiotomy is not a normal part of the puerperium we should
be making every effort to avoid it. Pain interferes with the
mother's enjoyment of her baby and there is no doubt that
early feeding problems arise because the mother cannot find
a comfortable position.

The second stage of labor should be conducted with the
objective of retaining an intact perineum -- or at most only
minimal lacerations.

The most important factors in making this likely are a
peaceful atmosphere, education of the mother, self control
and skillful verbal encouragement on the part of whoever is
delivering the baby.

A calm and unhurried atmosphere with a comfortable and
confident woman can greatly affect the degree of relaxation
and elasticity of the perineum -- whereas, if there is
tension, anxiety and hurry it is inevitable that this will
also be reflected.

It is the responsibility of whoever is conducting the
delivery to create a relaxed and emotionally supportive
environment for birth.

Previous education of the woman and her partner about
the mechanism of the second stage will make a great
contribution, but she still needs constant reassurance as
the second stage proceeds. Women who are having second
babies also need to be warned before the second stage begins
about the quality of the sensations they are going to feel.
This is particularly important if they have had a forceps
delivery or an epidural anesthetic. If this is not done they
may lose control and consequently damage their perineums.

There is much to be gained by allowing the second stage
of labor to proceed without active encouragement. The
involuntary expulsive efforts of the woman combined with the
uterine contractions will in most circumstances push the
presenting part down to the perineum without any great
effort on the woman's part. This practice also prevents the
possibility of mistakenly urging a woman to push against a
cervix that is not yet fully dilated. To do this may indeed
cause a future prolapse.

As the perineum begins to stretch, so will the
contractions become stronger and the woman begins to make a
voluntary expulsive effort. It is possible, in fact, to
manage a second stage without ever using the word "push."
This does not mean that one must stand silently by. Verbal
encouragement can play a very important part. It is easy to
note, for instance, when the woman contracts her anus during

contractions. There are two common causes for this both of which can be dealt with verbally. One is that she is afraid she will soil the bed. Recognizing this, and explaining it will not matter if she does, may be very helpful. The other is the burning sensation that is felt as the head starts moving more rapidly just before numbing occurs. Reassurance that she is not splitting at this time will be very welcome and reduce anxiety. One instruction that should not be given is to bear down as though constipated. Though the woman does feel great pressure on the rectum, using this command tends to lead to effort in the wrong direction — down and out rather than round and out.

There is often a period in a woman having a baby when she becomes disheartened and refuses to believe that she is making any progress. Encouraging the partner to see the presenting part and reporting back can be helpful. So too can be the use of a mirror, which allows a woman to see for herself and very often encourages good effort in the right direction. Some women like to feel the head with their fingers while it is still inside the vagina and derive renewed enthusiasm from this.

The position the woman adopts is of great importance. She should be so well supported that between contractions she can relax completely. She may be lying on her side or her back. In both positions her shoulders should be higher than her buttocks. Pushing when lying flat gives the woman an almost impossible task to perform. If she is on her back she may find it difficult to know what to do with her legs. Well prepared women may be able to drop their knees apart, placing their feet near their buttocks and rolling them out. An alternative is to encourage the woman to raise her feet off the bed by placing her hands around or under her knees. This prevents her from pushing against the bed with her feet which causes contractions of the pelvic floor. Pelvic floor contractions can also be caused by the attendants holding her legs with their hands under her feet, or by resting them against their bodies.

The woman will maintain control much better if she has not received Pethidine (Demerol) near the end of the first stage. Equally important, inhalational analgesia continued into the second stage may cause problems. The woman may imagine that the improvement in the quality of the contractions is due to the analgesia and be reluctant to try without. She should be encouraged to do so. In almost all cases she will manage perfectly well and become more alert and cooperative. Instrumental delivery can become necessary simply because of the effects of inhalational analgesia. The second stage is often painless although dramatic and yet still many members of the medical profession think that it is the most painful period of labor! Rapport between the midwife or doctor and the woman can be such that complete control of the delivery can be achieved verbally. But in many cases, manual control will also be required but should be achieved while causing as little discomfort to the woman as possible. Excessive pressure on the dilated anus causes uncontrolled contractions of the pelvic floor. This may result from a pad held too firmly or pressure from a hand. It is possible, by resting an outstretched hand gently on the distended perineum, to anticipate the crowning of the head by feeling the parietal bones moving past the fingers. If, at this time, extra control is required, steady pressure can be applied to the emerging head. Once the head has been safely delivered, great care must be taken with the delivery of the posterior shoulder — loss of control at this point could result in the only damage to the perineum occurring at this late stage.

Of course, throughout the second stage routine observations will be made. The condition of the woman and the fetus will be monitored and medical aid sought if progress is not consistent. These are necessary procedures, but they must not take precedence over other valuable skills required by the midwife or obstetrician which enables them to conduct the delivery with the perineum intact.

REFERENCES

1. DELEE J.B. The prophylactic forceps operation. Am J Obstet Gynecol 1:34-44, 1920.

2. CALDEYRO-BARCIA R. The influence of maternal bearing-down efforts during the second stage on fetal well-being. Birth Fam J 6:17-21, 1979. (Reprinted in this volume.)

3. BEYNON C.L. The normal second stage of labour — a plea for reform in its conduct. J Obstet Gynaecol Br Commonw 65(4):815, 1957. (Reprinted in this volume.)

7. The Management of Labor: An Obstetrician's View.

Ian Hoult, M.R.C.O.G., F.Aust.C.O.G.

Helping a woman to deliver without an episiotomy is not just a question of avoiding an incision. It is a matter of helping her coordinate pushing with spontaneous rhythms of her body so that she can actively give birth instead of engaging in a desperate race to get the baby out in as short a time as possible. The perineum is frequently subject to excessive strain because the laboring woman is urged to bear down harder, regardless of the strength of that particular contraction and whether or not she has a desire to push with it. Here an Australian specialist obstetrician working in a smaller country hospital maternity unit, gives his views on the conduct of the second stage, the way episiotomy should be done and subsequent care of the wound.

The operation of making and repairing an episiotomy has a definite place in the management of labor but like any other operative procedure, it is important to adhere to the indications for the operation and to be very aware of the risks and pitfalls.

Every practicing obstetrician knows of the distinctions between normal and abnormal labors and all of the former should be able to be delivered without the need for an episiotomy. The writer does not consider a simple mid-line perineal tear more harmful nor more difficult to repair than an episiotomy.

INDICATIONS FOR EPISIOTOMY

The need for an episiotomy should only arise in one or more of the following situations:

1. When delivery of the head is progressing at a rate or in a manner which will seriously tear the perineum or introital tissues and not allow time for the normal gentle stretching. This sort of situation may be encountered when the occiput is posterior, the presentation is compound or the delivery is uncontrolled and precipitant. The first consideration is to try to correct the problem itself so that normal perineal stretching can occur, but this may not always be possible.

2. Forceps deliveries and breech deliveries are very stylistic maneuvers but most obstetricians include episiotomy.

3. Prolonged delay with the head crowning but obstructed by a "tight perineum." This tends to be the commonest indication and is undoubtedly the area in which the biggest gains can be made by someone wanting to reduce

the episiotomy rate. This is the group of women who can be spared episiotomy by change of posture, a non-violent second stage and allowing for gentle stretching.

4. An emergency requires immediate delivery with the presenting part on view -- e.g., imminent eclampsia, fetal distress.

5. Previous vaginal, bladder and fistula repair operations, although of course many of these women are delivered by cesarean section.

If a previous episiotomy repair is ragged, uncomfortable and in need of repair it is usually appropriate to make a new episiotomy so as to enable one to clean up the edges and tissue of the previous scar. It is important to get it right the second time!

Having a list of "indications," it is important to remember that each episiotomy must be judged necessary on the merits of the case, alternative solutions having been rejected. Undoubtedly many episiotomies are performed because it is felt that something "has to be done," that routines must be adhered to or even worse, because of the impatience of the attending staff.

A previous episiotomy or tear is not necessarily an indication for a repeat operation although it behooves the attendant to consider the matter carefully, particularly in regard to the relative sizes of the infants and the rate of descent of the head. Furthermore, not all women being delivered of their first-born need an episiotomy.

REDUCING THE NEED FOR EPISIOTOMY

An enlightened attitude on the subject of episiotomy can really only come as part of a more sympathetic approach to the whole concept of childbirth. This ideally will be shared in its essentials by the mother, father and attendants.

The approach begins with antenatal consideration of the pelvic floor and perineal muscles. It is more important that the mother learn that these muscles will help her control second stage than that they should be "strong." Antenatal education needs to prepare women thoroughly on the control necessary as the head crowns because often only the clearest of instructions are remembered during the flurry of late second stage. Undoubtedly most women fear that perineal distention will be unbearably painful and the use of films, photos and other mothers' experiences should be used to counter this.

During the first stage of labor, correct posture and analgesia are important. Walking or sitting as distinct from lying down keeps the presenting part well on the cervix and descending in the pelvis. The recumbent position tends to make the mother a patient. It puts her in a posture of submission from which she is less able to contribute and be active. Judicious use of analgesia is important. Used incorrectly, analgesic drugs can result in loss of control by the mother. On the other hand, used appropriately if indicated and requested by the mother, analgesia may give her the brief rest she may need. Epidural analgesia and other forms of regional block greatly decrease the chances of spontaneous delivery without episiotomy. This is thought to be due to the loss of the reflex urge to push and paralysis of the pelvic floor muscles.

In the second stage of labor, posture is important. The mother should be in the position that she finds most suitable for pushing which does not result in appreciable changes in the fetal heart rate. Lying flat on the back should be avoided as the weight of the pregnant uterus can very materially affect the maternal (and hence placental) circulation. The left lateral, pillow-propped up, squatting and knee-chest positions are among many that different women find best.

The mother needs someone she trusts immediately at hand to assist keeping her mind to the task. Quiet, non-interfering efficiency and informed explanation and discussion are required of the attending staff.

Pushing should be allowed to come as the natural response in the reflex resulting from the descent of the head during each contraction. This method is quite distinct from the usual practice of giving the command "push" at the beginning of each contraction and repeating the command right through while the patient's breath is held and her face blue. This "natural" or, more correctly, "responding" push need not be violent. Pushing in a comfortable position will result in the steady descent of the vertex onto the perineum where the urge to push becomes more demanding and often somewhat painful as distention occurs. It is at this stage that a little gentle thinning of the fourchette (the posterior rim of the maternal opening at this stage) with a gloved finger lubricated with a little oil or local anesthetic jelly can help the perineum stretch.

Finally remember that the fetal head comes through the introitus by flexion and if extension occurs a wider diameter will come through and increase the chances of a tear. Flexion is maintained by knowing the position of the occiput and encouraging that part of the head to come through before the parts more anterior to it. Once the head is delivered it is important to take care getting the shoulders across the perineum. One should wait for a contraction and the woman's urge to push before delivering the shoulders, unless medical urgency dictates haste. It is common for the posterior shoulder to make a small posterior vaginal laceration if the delivery of the shoulder is effected by traction.

MAKING AN EPISIOTOMY

The episiotomy itself has several fine points worthy of discussion. It is vital that the scissors are good instruments -- they must be able to make the necessary cut in a single movement. More than one cut with the episiotomy scissors usually increases the discomfort of the incision and scar and tends to make it ragged. Analgesia is necessary and if a local anesthetic agent (usually 1% Lignocaine) is used, it is important to wait the necessary period of time to allow the anesthetic to work before checking its effectiveness and proceeding with the operation. Most women benefit from a brief explanation of the need for an episiotomy. Ideally antenatal education and discussion on the subject will enable a quick and mutually satisfactory decision to be made at the time.

The question of informed consent to perform episiotomy is rarely considered. The relationship between medical workers and the law is not the same in the U.S.A., Great Britain, Australia and other countries. Nevertheless, presumably the principles of the relationship have certain things in common.

Informed consent as a principle has two aspects. Firstly it is a system of "protection" of the person doing something to a patient. But far more importantly it involves the patient's right of self-determination and autonomy which stem from political notions of the importance of the individual.

Now, the writer does not have a woman sign a form of consent for episiotomy for two reasons. Firstly it would be cumbersome and would imply that I were trying to protect myself legally. But more importantly, it would distract from the real purpose of my seeking her consent -- the attempt to find common ground with her expectations, even if this means falling somewhat short of them. I always aim to have a knowledge of a woman's feelings about episiotomy. If I feel that the operation is indicated I make a brief but precise explanation and then look for the woman's implied consent.

The presenting part should be well down and really stretching the perineum before making the episiotomy. If the head is only just coming into view and the perineum beginning to distend, episiotomy at this stage will only result in a lot of bleeding, anxiety, discomfort, bruising and wound infection.

It is imperative that the incision begin in the middle of the posterior edge of the introitus. Thereafter the various techniques all have their proponents. The mid-line episiotomy bleeds less and heals much better.

Whatever technique is used, an episiotomy that begins other than in the middle of the fourchette is likely to give a very uncomfortable step in the healed wound which will subsequently cause discomfort during intercourse.

The writer has come to the opinion that the mid-line episiotomy is far more preferable than the medio-lateral and J-shaped procedures. Second degree extension does occur from time to time and even third degree to include the mucosa of the anal canal. Nevertheless, repair with care still gives excellent results. The medio-lateral operations frequently give an uncomfortable and unsightly long-term scar.

The introitus, perineum and indeed the whole vagina are often best inspected before delivery of the placenta because the placenta dams back uterine blood and hence usually allows for a better view. Always take special care inspecting the para-urethral tissues, the labia minora and deep in the vagina.

REPAIRING AN EPISIOTOMY

The episiotomy should be repaired by the person who made the incision. No time should be lost in making the repair as the longer a surgical wound is left open, the greater the chance of wound infection. The writer rarely has a woman put in the lithotomy position for perineal suture -- it is really only required for complicated repairs.

Inspection of the wound should define its limits and landmarks and extensions up the vagina and toward the rectum noted. The apex of the episiotomy or the uppermost end of its extension should be firmly secured to achieve hemostasis. If the anal sphincter has been divided it should be reconstructed with interrupted sutures.

An episiotomy is usually closed in layers with continuous catgut to the vaginal skin making sure that the landmarks (especially carunculae myrtiformes) are brought together from both sides of the incision. The deep tissues of the perineum are brought together using chromic catgut. These sutures normally achieve hemostasis. Finally the perineal skin can be closed with interrupted non-absorbable sutures such as silk. Done with care, a chromic catgut subcuticular suture gives a neat, closed and perhaps more comfortable episiotomy wound. Polyglycolic acid sutures give even better results (in terms of pain and edema) than chromic catgut.

At the end of every episiotomy repair it is a good rule to examine the vagina to exclude ongoing bleeding and to check that no pack or other foreign body has been left there. A simple digital rectum examination checks that none of the sutures has gone into the rectum and that the anal sphincter has substance to it all the way around.

Two further generalizations concern speed and exactness. All other things being equal, a short operation is less likely to get infected than a long one and also hurts less. A common error is to be too particular about getting every little skin fold aligned to its partner on the other side of the wound. If taken too far the wound becomes full of catgut which frequently causes wound breakdown. With the main landmarks as guides an episiotomy should be closed with just a few well placed sutures rather than many lengths of catgut in every corner.

The description above includes the various methods and principles taught to the writer in his training. What follows describes his preferred technique.

Lignocaine 1% local anesthetic without adrenalin is used to infiltrate the stretched perineum. A mid-line episiotomy is always preferred. If the third stage is delayed, repair of the episiotomy is commenced while waiting.

If the anal sphincter is damaged, it is repaired with a single suture. The vaginal skin is not sutured. The deep tissues of the perineum are brought together using sutures with only moderate suture-tissue tension (not tight!). These sutures lie just deep to the vaginal and external skin. Usually three or four such sutures close the average episiotomy. Of special importance is the avoidance of any sutures at the posterior introital edge. The avoidance of sutures in the skin makes for a comfortable, fast-healing non-infected wound.

AFTERCARE

A healing episiotomy hurts and most women require some analgesia. An ice pack (ice chips in a latex disposable glove) for the first twenty-four hours has a numbing effect and reduces bruising and swelling. The wound should be kept clean and dry and the bidet is ideal for this. Topical heat using a ray lamp aids healing and helps keep the wound dry. Equally a hair-dryer is very effective at keeping the wound dry.

Intercourse will not damage the repair once it is comfortable which is usually after two weeks. If the introitus has been narrowed by the repair, gentle digital dilatation and intercourse is far preferable to a repeat operation. The husband should be made aware of the presence of the episiotomy wound and the need for gentleness while his wife is returning to full sexual ability.

If the wound should open or break down completely, one should advise that the wound be left to granulate and subsequently heal. Secondary suture is generally to be avoided as healing will be poor. Should it be necessary, granulating and infected tissue should be excised and a new closure made using non-absorbable sutures.

Episiotomy is a technical procedure with considerable psychological consequences. There are indications for its use, but to avoid performing episiotomy in every case it is necessary to aim for women to deliver themselves spontaneously with a controlled second stage. The co-ordination required to achieve this comes from antenatal education and cooperation from the attendants during labor. Ignorance about what is happening to her together with unnecessary arrogance, anxiety or haste on behalf of the attendants leads to a train of problems and acts of interference, one of which is an unnecessary episiotomy.

8. Birth Over the Intact Perineum: A Clinical Approach.

David Priver, M.D.

In the United States, episiotomy is performed on almost all primigravidas and most multigravidas. Medical schools teach that episiotomy is the only way to preserve and protect the perineum. Here, an American obstetrician who has rejected this conventional practice, describes his rationale and management techniques to maintain an intact perineum.

The prevalent view that routine episiotomy serves to reduce trauma to maternal tissues has never been substantiated by scientific analysis, and has been accepted by the obstetrical community largely on faith. We have all heard the dire warnings that lack of episiotomy predisposes to all manner of future anatomic and sexual disorders, but have we ever questioned the validity of these fears? What of other countries where episiotomy is rarely practiced? There is certainly no report of higher incidences of uterine prolapse, cystocele, and the like in these countries. At a time when consumers are questioning nearly every aspect of their medical care, it behooves us to reevaluate the issue of episiotomy so that we may provide our patients with safe, sound, and supportive medical care.

Having studied this issue over the past few years, I would submit that relatively few healthy, informed, secure, and motivated women need episiotomy. If the matter is approached logically and sensibly, most patients are able to exercise the control necessary to give birth to their babies in a gradual, controlled fashion which rarely requires any operative intervention. In this article, I will set forward the approach which I have used sucessfully for several years. I hope that by doing so, interest will be generated in reevaluating many of the management techniques used in obstetrics today, especially those employed in the second stage of labor.

While most of us still feel that the hospital is the soundest location for birth, there can be no doubt that many women can bear the stresses of labor quite nicely without analgesia or anesthesia or many of the other time-honored obstetrical interventions. If women are motivated to prepare physically and emotionally for childbirth and are permitted by their attendants to utilize sound "physiologic" techniques in labor, there is usually no need to employ such tools as forceps, episiotomy, and lithotomy position. These tools, potentially valuable as they may be, should be reserved for the "high-risk" or anesthetized patient. With this in mind, let us now consider how we may go about providing care to the low-risk laboring woman who is desirous of avoiding episiotomy. We shall begin by considering prenatal factors and then proceed to the major emphasis on intrapartum techniques, followed by a brief discussion of postpartum considerations.

I. PRENATAL FACTORS

Motivation. The single most significant factor in determining the outcome of this effort is probably the degree of motivation involved. This applies to both the patient and the physician. They must both feel that the extra preparation and time involved is worthwhile, otherwise either or both may find it too easy to abandon the effort. On the other hand, once the practitioner has become experienced and confident with the technique, he may wish to use it on all of his patients. We must remember that there will always be patients to whom the issue of episiotomy is of little importance. For them it is better to do routine episiotomy since they will probably not prepare themselves prepartum and not exercise postpartum, and the results are likely to be poor.

Physical Conditioning. Birth over the intact perineum requires a great deal of muscular control, especially of the pelvic floor. Also, the woman may need to utilize several positions requiring her to support much or all of her weight during second stage. Accordingly, patients should be encouraged to begin fairly vigorous exercises designed to strengthen muscles of the low back, thighs, and pelvic floor no later than the end of the fifth month. Kegel exercises and maintaining of squatting positions are very helpful.

Nutrition. It should be obvious that any birth method involving strength and stamina will require a nutritional program providing adequate sources of protein and energy. A minimum of 80 grams of protein and 2,500 calories per day should provide for adequate fetal growth and maternal energy needs.

Relaxation and Stress Reduction. The ability to voluntarily relax skeletal muscles is one of the most critical factors in determining the success of this effort. This is true for two major reasons. First, it has been amply documented that much of the pain of labor relates to skeletal muscle contraction. If a laboring woman can respond to contractions by reducing muscle tension, she can substantially reduce her level of discomfort. Secondly, the expulsion of the head is often hindered by contraction of the levatores. In a sense, the patient is fearful of relaxing these muscles, and must be carefully taught and encouraged to do so. She must be reassured that she will not be injured in the process and that the tissues are capable of adequate stretching. Gentle encouragement to "open up" and to "let go" can be very helpful. I continue to find it nearly astonishing how much more quickly and smoothly the birth proceeds when the patient manages to master this technique. Prenatal perineal massage, if done correctly, can help the patient learn how to do this; this will be discussed in more detail later.

Muscle relaxation is best facilitated when the woman is able to labor under conditions of minimal psychic stress. In addition, it is well recognized that a stressed patient, producing and releasing adrenaline, tends to labor slowly and poorly due to the inhibitory effects of adrenaline on the strength of uterine contractions. An additional, and perhaps more ominous, effect is vasoconstriction with its potential for decreased placental blood flow and fetal hypoxia. For all these reasons, it is important to provide a secure and comfortable environment and to avoid unnecessary intrusions into the patient's privacy. If the patient can know before labor that efforts will be made to ensure these conditions, she will tend to labor more efficiently.

Communication and Education. None of what we have discussed so far and will be discussing hence is of any value whatever unless it can be effectively conveyed to the patient. The overall importance of unbiased and knowledgeable prenatal education simply cannot be overstated. One of the greatest obstacles to physiologic birth care is simple lack of knowledge that such a thing even exists. Women often express amazement to find that labor and birth can be effectively and comfortably carried out without routine epidurals, forceps, and episiotomy. With the unfortunate trend toward hospital-based childbirth classes in this country, however, the teaching curricula are often prescribed and inhibited by those who do not wish to have their routines upset or their rationales questioned. How many hospital-based childbirth classes presently teach methods of avoidance of episiotomy? What would be the likely fate of an instructor who wished to introduce this concept? We hope the near future will see more independent childbirth teaching as well as a resumption by the caring obstetrician to recapture his role of teacher as well as healer.

Perineal Massage. As part of a continuing effort to become more familiar and comfortable with her body, the pregnant woman should begin frequent perineal massage by the sixth or seventh month. There are many benefits to perineal massage. If carried out using a topical form of vitamin E, the perineal skin may gain much-needed elasticity. Also, the woman can become accustomed to pressure sensations in this area similar to what she will encounter during labor. An especially helpful technique is to have her partner insert two fingers into the vagina and depress the levator muscles, much the way the baby's head will do during labor. The patient can thus learn the technique of voluntarily relaxing these muscles against pressure, a critically important ability during birth. (See Appendix A for complete instructions in prenatal perineal massage.)

II.   INTRAPARTUM TECHNIQUES

Risk Status. Planned avoidance of episiotomy, at least in the primigravida, is, by its very nature, a technique designed for low-risk birth situations. Entailing, as it does, a slower delivery and intermittent rather than continuous fetal monitoring, it would appear prudent to forego the efforts if any suspicion exists of maternal or fetal compromise. As a guideline (which certainly could be modified in the future as more experience is acquired) the following conditions should exist at the onset of labor:

1. Term pregnancy (or nearly so)
In order to avoid cerebral trauma in the premature fetus with its incompletely calcified cranium, the pregnancy should be at least 36 weeks by reliable clinical dating.

2. Normal FHR pattern
A 20 to 30 minute admitting monitoring strip should confirm a normal baseline rate with good short-term variability and no late decelerations or severe variable decelerations.

3. No identifiable medical or obstetrical complications

4. Vertex presentation
A vaginal breech delivery would not lend itself to this method since fairly expeditious delivery of the after-coming head is mandatory due to the potential hazard of umbilical cord obstruction.

Freedom of Movement During First Stage. Several studies have now made it clear that the first stage of labor is more efficient as well as less uncomfortable when carried out in upright, ambulatory positions.[1,2] Accordingly, the patient should be advised of this fact and encouraged to walk often and to rest in sitting positions. The commonly expressed fear of umbilical cord prolapse is yet another example of a time-honored obstetric belief which has never been documented. Intravenous lines may be used, if felt necessary, but should be used with portable IV poles. Fetal monitors also may be used as needed, but use should either be intermittent or should employ the newer telemetry instruments so that the patient can ambulate while being monitored.

Some OB units are reluctant to permit ambulation for fear of maternal injury in the event of a fall. For this reason, ambulation should be limited to patients judged not to be excessively fatigued, stressed, narcotized, or sedated. A companion should also be present if the nurse is not available. With the information we now have available regarding the obvious benefits of ambulation, all patients should be automatically ambulated unless specific orders to the contrary are received.

This approach will improve the chances of avoiding episiotomy by providing a smoother, less painful dilatation and descent, thereby enabling the patient to work more effectively with the demands of second stage labor.

Avoidance of Drugs Which Affect Neuromuscular Faculties. The effort to avoid episiotomy is largely dependent upon a patient who is alert, responsive, and able to assume comfortable, effective positions during labor. Narcotics and sedatives will quite obviously work against the woman's ability to concentrate and focus her efforts, at least in the short run. Patients should be prepared to utilize non-pharmacologic pain relief techniques before resorting to drugs. Physical methods such as heat, showers or baths, pressure, massage, breathing, relaxation, and position change can often be quite satisfactory, especially if the patient is working with calm and supportive birth companions.

Epidural anesthesia, while offering the advantages of safety, comfort, and muscle relaxation, should also be avoided if possible, due to its muscle-weakening effect. Once an epidural has been administered, the patient is confined to bed and cannot take advantage of helpful positions. Also, there is interference with reflexes, sensations, and pushing capability, all of which tend to reduce effectiveness and control in second stage.

It should be emphasized that no patient should ever be forced or even encouraged to suffer through an abnormally painful and stressful labor without analgesia. In addition to the dictates of simple human compassion, the importance of stress reduction and subsequent elimination of the hazards of excess adrenaline release vastly outweigh the need to avoid episiotomy!

Comfortable, Effective Position in Second Stage. Studies of birth techniques in other countries and cultures have demonstrated an overwhelming preference for squatting and similar positions during second stage.[3] It appears to be a position in which there is much mechanical advantage as well as a high degree of comfort and control. X-ray studies have confirmed that a woman in squatting position actually achieves a widening of her interspinous diameter by nearly a full centimeter and an increase in the surface area of the pelvic outlet of 30%.[4]

Unfortunately, there has been reluctance to utilize this position in this country for a variety of reasons. As mentioned earlier, the use of drugs and anesthetics in first stage largely eliminates the woman's ability to support herself. Also, the squatting position is simply not used for any other activities (unlike in third world countries), and is therefore quite unfamiliar to most American women. Some have expressed distaste for the position, apparently equating it with excretory functions, and feeling that it is not "ladylike." Just how "ladylike" the lithotomy position is is open to debate!

Regardless of one's emotional reaction to the squatting position, there can be no argument with its often astonishing effectiveness in resolving a difficult second stage and preserving the woman's strength for controlling the expulsion of the head. (See Appendix B on Teaching Squatting.)

Physiologic Pushing. It has been demonstrated that prolonged, forceful pushing associated with breath-holding can be deleterious to the fetus. Late decelerations are often associated with this effort. In addition, pushing efforts of this sort are extremely fatiguing for the mother. Also, the rapid stretching of vaginal tissue caused by this method may predispose to laceration rather than smooth dilatation. For these reasons, it is now recommended that pushing be carried out in a far more gentle manner. Instead of breath-holding, the mother is taught to keep the glottis open and permit a gradual release of air. Also, the push is kept relatively short, around 5-8 seconds, with the mother advised to stop, take another breath, and repeat, more or less in accord with her physiologic instincts.

While this method may prolong the second stage somewhat, it results in a less stressed mother and infant and thus permits second stage to be safely observed well beyond the arbitrary two hour time limit, so long as progress is seen and the FHTs are stable.

Expulsive Phase of Second Stage. At that point in the primiparous labor when crowning begins (and somewhat earlier in the multipara), is started what may be referred to as the "expulsive" phase. With the new sensations, physical relationships, and methods used, it should be thought of as a type of labor distinctly different from earlier second stage. The woman now reports a greater pushing urge as well as a "burning" sensation at the vulva and perineum. The fetal head has reached the perineum, and is beginning to extend. Obviously, this is the point where the most concentrated and critical efforts are needed if the perineum is to stretch smoothly and episiotomy avoided.

Massage of the perineum should be started in an effort to flatten, soften, and "iron" it. The examiner should also try to palpate the levator muscles if there is any indication that they are not being adequately relaxed. If excessive tension is found, the patient should be reminded of perineal relaxation and should try to voluntarily relax the muscles against the gentle examining fingers between contractions.

A warmed lubricating oil should be generously employed for this technique (e.g., almond or wheat germ oil). This improves comfort for the patient and enhances perineal softening. Some concerns have been expressed as to the potential for bacterial contamination from the oil, but no reports of infection related to its use have appeared. Similarly, some have raised fears that the baby could aspirate the oil, but this has also not been reported.

Along with massage, the use of hot, moist compresses held gently against the vulva and perineum provides for excellent comfort and relaxation. In general, the patients prefer as much heat as reasonably possible; no one has ever complained about the compresses being too hot! During the final few contractions, the woman will commonly complain of much burning in the periurethral and clitoral areas. Applying compresses in these locations is usually quite helpful and well received.

As in the earlier stages of labor, maternal position is quite critical. The position used to bring the head down to the perineum in early second stage will not necessarily be the most comfortable and effective at this point. Once again, the woman should be encouraged to try several positions if her present one seems uncomfortable or inefficient. Hands-and-knees position is frequently most effective as it tends to drop the head away from the sacrum and coccyx and also to reduce pressure against the perineum. At first thought, the 180-degree change in the orientation of the patient seems confusing to the attendant, but the birth is actually quite easy to manage as a little experience will quickly demonstrate. If the woman is fatigued or the birth is coming quite rapidly, lateral Sims position is an excellent alternative, although an additional assistant is needed to elevate the patient's upper leg.

One of the most critical features of the expulsive phase is the necessity to avoid any further pushing efforts. As the perineum is often paper-thin at this point, pushing would be very likely to cause a laceration. Therefore, the birth must be carried out as gradually as possible. This is accomplished by having the woman pant rapidly and shallowly. As her urge to push is quite strong, this technique requires intense "coaching." The coach should place himself closely face-to-face with the patient and breathe with her. He must encourage her to keep her eyes open and follow his lead. Although this is one of the most demanding points in the labor, it is fortunately quite short, as the patient should be taught well in advance.

It is also important to make efforts to keep the fetal head well flexed until the brow can be seen. This permits the occipito-frontal diameter to present rather than the larger occipito-bregmatic, thus reducing the amount of stretching required. This is in direct contradistinction to the Ritgen maneuver which calls for early extension of the head.

It is easy to see that all these techniques, taken together, result in a slower birth than most of us are used to. The patient should be told to expect the birth to take from 5 to 30 minutes longer when done this way. It is most important to maintain frequent surveillance of fetal heart tones during this time. If the heart rate drops to 90/min. or less, or if progress is poor, the mother's position should be changed. If either of these problems is not resolved within 5 minutes, one should abandon the technique and proceed immediately with episiotomy and delivery.

Delivery of Shoulders. It is not infrequent to accomplish the birth of the head with the perineum intact, only to have the shoulders cause a laceration. Great control must continue to be exercised until birth of the shoulders is completed. After checking for the umbilical cord, one should encourage the mother to push gently until the anterior shoulder is seen. (In a hands-and-knees birth, the posterior shoulder usually presents first.) If a large baby is anticipated, one should try to proceed with delivery of the arm before trying for the second shoulder. This avoids the added stretching required by having both shoulders at the vulva simultaneously. As the second shoulder is born, one should place the flat of the hand against the perineum for support.

III. POST PARTUM

Examination. If the mother's and baby's conditions are normal and stable, the examination can be delayed until after cutting the cord, delivery of the placenta, and immediate maternal-infant bonding. Usually, the infant may remain in the mother's arms during the exam. In the absence of forceps, there is usually no need to visually inspect the cervix, and manual exploration of the uterus should be avoided unless there is strong evidence of retained placental tissue, in which case the exam should probably be done in the delivery room under anesthesia with antibiotic coverage.

Close inspection of the periurethral area, perineum, and vaginal walls is imperative, but must be done very gently. If the exam is negative, but bleeding is persisting with the uterus well contracted, it is mandatory to put the patient in lithotomy and examine with adequate lighting and sedation, if necessary.

Suture Repair. In 30 to 40% of these cases, there are noticeable abrasions present. In general, if they are not bleeding, they do not have to be repaired. Some amount of suturing will be required in about half of these instances (i.e., 50% of the patients with abrasions, or 15-20% of all non-episiotomy patients). Presumably, these percentages will decrease as more experience is gained with the techniques.

Contrary to popular obstetrical belief, the few lacerations which do occur tend to be smooth, even, and quite easy to repair. The gradual nature of the birth usually restricts tears to the midline of the perineum, much similar to a small episiotomy. This is especially true of the woman attempting this method who has had a previous episiotomy.

Due to the longer second stage and greater pressure against the perineum, it is advisable to use an ice pack after delivery even if no laceration or repair is involved.

Recovery. As soon as perineal edema is reduced (4 to 5 days), the patient should resume Kegel exercises. She should know in advance that the extra stretching involved in this approach will require a vigorous effort at re-establishing perineal muscle tone. Although some amount of "gaping" is not unusual at first, the patient should be reassured that full recovery should occur by no later than 8 to 10 weeks post partum. An interim exam at 3 to 4 weeks can serve to evaluate progress and to determine if more vigorous exercise is needed.

CONCLUSION

The methods described in this paper are designed to permit the healthy, well-motivated woman to have a chance at delivering over an intact perineum. They are based on concepts of physiology which require an alert and controlled patient working with a supportive physician, and employing effective positions. Even under all these optimal conditions, it will often not be appropriate to use the methods for a variety of reasons. Patients need to be educated as to the availability of this approach, but should be strongly dissuaded from focusing on it as the most important aspect of a "good" birth experience. One must realize, after all, that our ultimate objective remains the good health of the mother and baby, and this may preclude the extra time and effort required to give birth in this manner.

Having said this, however, I would hope that all practicing obstetricians would take the time to learn these methods. They will serve as a valuable addition to our armament of skills, and will enable us to offer a more wide-ranging and flexible service to our patients. I also hope these skills will also encourage us to more readily appreciate and utilize the marvelous array of physiologic techniques at our disposal to help solve many obstetrical problems.

REFERENCES

1. Mendez-Bauer C, et al. Effects of standing position on spontaneous uterine contractility and other aspects of labor. J Perinatal Med 3:89, 1975.

2. Flynn AM, et al. Ambulation in labour. Br Med J 2:591, 1978.

3. Englemann George. Labor Among Primitive Peoples, 1882. Reprinted 1977: AMS Press Inc. N.Y.

4. Russell JGB. Moulding of the pelvic outlet. J Obstet Gynaecol Br Commonw 76:817, 1969.

5. Caldeyro-Barcia R. The influence of maternal bearing-down efforts during second stage on fetal well-being. Birth Family J 6(1):17, 1979. (Reprinted in this volume.)

9. Benefits and Risks of Episiotomy.

David Banta, M.D. and Stephen B. Thacker, M.D.

(This paper first appeared in Birth: Issues in Perinatal Care and Education 9(1):25-30, Spring 82, and is reprinted here with permission.)

Almost all nulliparas and most multiparas in North America have episiotomies. In seeking the rationale for this, two American epidemiologists conducted a vast survey of the English medical literature as far back as 1860. Here they report their findings.

This paper is based on an intensive review of the scientific literature on the risks and benefits of episiotomy, the surgical enlargement of the vaginal orifice during labor or delivery.[41,42] Why were we concerned about episiotomy? First, medical technologies (drugs, devices, and medical/surgical procedures used in medical care) have been increasingly questioned during the past five years. This questioning has focused primarily on new, capital-intensive technology such as computerized axial tomography (the CAT scanner). Generally, however, we have come to realize that the primary problem is not that of new capital-intensive technology. Rather it is the frequent use of low-capital procedures such as episiotomy that are done at great expense for uncertain benefit. Second, we had previously carried out a similar literature review on electronic fetal monitoring,[2,3] which stimulated our interest in obstetric care. For the last five to ten years the use of technology in obstetrical practice has been questioned as much as in any medical discipline. In addition to electronic fetal monitoring, criticisms have been leveled at the inappropriate use of cesarean section,[31] induction of labor,[15] perineal shaving[27] and obstetric anesthesia.[8] Consequently, we began to think in terms of looking at an obstetrical practice that was a low-capital procedure.

Perineotomy is actually the technical term for the procedure described above as episiotomy, but we are following the usual practice of calling the procedure an episiotomy. Today, there are two major ways to carry out an episiotomy: either the medio-lateral incision, which is more frequent in other countries such as England, or the median incision, which is generally preferred in the United States (Figure 1). There are advantages and disadvantages to each approach, all fairly well supported by clinical experience.[10,17,22,39] The median incision is easier to repair, less painful, and associated with less loss of blood. However, the medio-lateral incision is less

frequently associated with extension of the episiotomy into
the anal sphincter and rectum.

Episiotomy is the second most common surgical procedure
done in the United States after cutting the umbilical
cord.[33] The routine use of episiotomy is rarely questioned
in the medical literature, although there are critical
articles in the nurse-midwifery literature.[18] The practice
of episiotomy has also been questioned in the lay literature
and, in fact, conversations with the editors of Our Bodies,
Ourselves were a stimulus to this work.

LITERATURE REVIEW

The process by which we obtained information on
episiotomy is itself of some interest. The review began with
an examination of information found in the MEDLINE system, a
computerized listing of a large portion of the world's
medical literature. Unfortunately, this system provided no
information on episiotomy prior to 1968. Essentially all of
the articles available in MEDLINE were reports of randomized
controlled clinical trials of the relative efficacies of
pain medications using episiotomy pain as a standard. We
found it rather peculiar that there were no articles about
pain as it relates to episiotomy, but a number of reports
having to do with the treatment of pain using episiotomy as
a model.[6] We also reviewed published bibliographies from
various sources such as other articles and textbooks.
Eventually, we reviewed published indexes of the medical
literature back to 1860 to identify any papers that might
deal with episiotomy, not only to look for data, but also to
try to understand the historical factors that led to the
widespread use of this procedure. It was soon apparent that
there were little scientific data to support the widespread
use of episiotomy. Indeed, if one restricts the definition
of scientific data to that which is obtained from a
randomized controlled clinical trial, there were no data
to support the use of episiotomy. Nevertheless, the use of
episiotomy appears justified in selected clinical
situations, such as impending laceration (or tear) and in
conjunction with the application of forceps. Therefore, we
confined ourselves to examining the use of episiotomy
without specific indications for its use (sometimes called
"routine" episiotomy).

There is a fairly large number of clinical studies
which include data on episiotomy, but except for the
analgesia studies mentioned previously, these reports are
very old and scientifically inadequate. We reviewed over 400
articles and decided that over 150 of them were totally
without merit, leaving nearly 250 articles in our final
bibliography.

While there are limitations to this kind of literature review, it can tell one something about the scientific basis for decision-making in medicine. Such a review cannot provide proof of efficacy (benefit) and safety. Still, the literature is the repository of scientific knowledge, so we think that it does tell a lot about why a practice was begun or continues to be done. Our analysis is biased by a belief in solid epidemiologic principles and a philosophical belief that technology (particularly technology that is associated with significant risk) should not be used without good evidence of benefit. Many physicians feel that clinical experience provides an adequate basis for good practice and would simply disagree with our position regarding necessity of evidence.

HISTORICAL PERSPECTIVE

Ould first used the perineal incision in 1742 to facilitate difficult deliveries. But his procedure found little acceptance until the late 1800s and early 1900s, in part because anesthesia was not available and infection rates were so high that surgery was considered to be a very serious undertaking.[37] Beginning in the late 1800s, an increasing number of physicians advocated episiotomy for certain complicated pregnancies, but resistance to the procedure persisted until the strong advocacy of two prominent obstetricians, Pomeroy[38] and DeLee.[20] The acceptance of episiotomy paralleled the shift to hospital delivery. In 1930, 25 percent of women delivered in the hospital; by 1945 this figure increased to over 70 percent.[43] In 1979, 62.5 percent of deliveries in the United States were estimated to include an episiotomy.[33] Episiotomy data by parity, however, are not available. Individual institutions report episiotomy rates of 80-90 percent or more for primiparous women and perhaps 50 percent for multiparas.

Aside from the poor quality of the medical literature, there is a number of factors that make it difficult to assess episiotomy. First, the changes in parity have been rather remarkable over the last few decades. Among women born in 1850, 40 percent had seven or more deliveries.[11] Only 21 percent of women in the 1929 cohort had five or more children. It appears that in the 1945 cohort only 5 percent of women will have five or more deliveries.[12] Therefore, in considering the complications and possible benefits of episiotomy, especially concerning pelvic damage, this reduction in numbers of children born is probably much more important than episiotomy.

BENEFITS OF EPISIOTOMY

There are four reported benefits of episiotomy.[39]
First, it is asserted that a clean, straight incision is
easier to repair, and that it heals better than a laceration
or tear. Second, it is claimed that there are fewer
third-degree lacerations following episiotomy. Third, it is
stated that episiotomy prevents fetal brain injury because
it reduces the pressure of the fetal head on the pelvic
floor. Fourth, episiotomy is said to shorten the second
stage of labor which, in turn, helps to prevent damage to
the pelvic floor.

Ease of Repair

It is true that a clean, surgical incision is easier to
repair than a contaminated, irregular laceration. In such
circumstances healing of episiotomy is no doubt more rapid.
The question in relation to episiotomy, however, is first
how frequently such a clear-cut situation pertains and then,
in a properly designed study, what outcomes are observed.
Current opinion is based on clinical impressions, not on
data from studies of women undergoing labor and delivery.
There is, of course, the question as to how many repairs are
even necessary with and without an episiotomy. Obviously, if
every woman undergoes an episiotomy, repair is required.
Yet, a sizable number of women who do not undergo episiotomy
do not require surgical repair following delivery, up to 50
percent in some studies.[9,19,24] Is the pain and discomfort
resulting from these seemingly unnecessary procedures
warranted? Although this question is not specifically
addressed in the medical literature, one can reasonably ask
for another justification for episiotomy.

Fewer Third-degree Lacerations

Let us then consider the question of third-degree
laceration, an incision or tearing of tissue that extends
into the anus or rectum. None of the published studies is
controlled, and some are very old (Table 1). For what these
data are worth, they certainly do not provide convincing
evidence that episiotomy prevents third-degree laceration.
The data do seem to indicate that fewer third-degree
lacerations occur following medio-lateral episiotomy, but
even this conclusion is uncertain because of poor study
designs. Three studies of episiotomy were controlled, but
interpretation is complicated both by serious problems with
the selection or nature of the controls, and the conflicting
evidence.[9,16,37] Again, these studies give no clear
indication that episiotomy prevents third-degree laceration.

TABLE I

Percentage of women having an episiotomy complicated by third-degree lacerations, by type of incision, 33 studies, 1919–1980.

Type	No. of Studies	Third-Degree Lacerations	
		Range (%)	Weighted Average (%)
Episiotomy			
Midline	15	0.2 – 23.9	3.6
Mediolateral	6	0.0 – 9.0	0.6
Unspecified	5	0.0 – 17.2	4.0
No Episiotomy	7	0.0 – 6.4	2.0

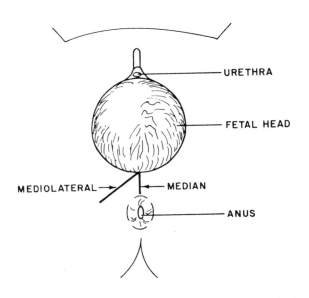

Figure I. Median and Mediolateral Episiotomies

It is also evident from these data that episiotomies
sometimes tear further and can extend into the rectum.

Prevention of Fetal Brain Damage

There are simply no data to evaluate the effectiveness
of episiotomy in preventing fetal brain damage. Extensive
studies suggest that most factors leading to cerebral palsy
and severe mental retardation precede labor and
delivery.[34,35,36] The only other evidence concerning this
alleged benefit of episiotomy is indirect and is related to
the length of the second stage of labor. There are several
practices that unquestionably shorten the second stage,
including episiotomy, the use of forceps, and the use of
oxytocin. Episiotomy seems to shorten the second stage of
labor by 15 to 30 minutes.[32,42] A shortened second stage
may decrease the risk of intrapartum fetal asphyxia and,
consequently, decrease the risk of brain damage to the
infant. However, active pushing, which is one of the ways of
speeding labor, causes fetal hypoxia.[13] Hence, speeding
labor may also increase the risk of brain damage.

An important study of the second stage of labor
compared the effects on pregnancy outcome for 100 women who
were not urged to push to 393 who were.[5] These groups were
not randomly selected; rather, selection was solely a result
of physician preference, so the results must be interpreted
with caution. In the non-pushing group, 6 percent of women
required forceps to complete delivery, compared to 11.9
percent in the other group. A total of 39 percent who were
not urged to push had a laceration or episiotomy that
required repair, compared to 63 percent in the other group.
These data, then, suggest that active pushing may also
result in postpartum complications for the mother.

Prevention of Pelvic Relaxation

Pelvic relaxation has been estimated to occur in up to
10 percent of deliveries, but there really are no good
epidemiological data concerning the rate of pelvic
relaxation in the population of childbearing women and there
is no study with a follow-up of longer than six months.[21]
There have been three controlled studies of pelvic
relaxation and its relationship to episiotomy.[1,9,37] Two
studies, done over 45 years ago, showed decreased pelvic
damage among women undergoing episiotomy.[1,37] However, the
selection of control groups in these two studies was
seriously biased, making interpretation of the studies
difficult. A better controlled study reported in 1975 showed
equivalent outcomes, but has a small sample size.[9] Taken
together, these findings are inconclusive. Not only do they
have problems in methods, but they do not deal adequately

with current changes in childbearing practices. Preliminary results from a longitudinal evaluation of the pelvic tissues of women who did not have episiotomy show very low rates of relaxation.[14]

In summary, the data on benefits of episiotomy are very poor and offer no convincing argument to support the routine use of that procedure.

RISKS

On the other hand, there is no paper in the literature focusing on the risks associated with episiotomy. Virtually all of the data on pain were obtained from trials on pain medications, which had used episiotomy as a model.[6] There is clearly a difference in perception as to the magnitude and importance of post-episiotomy pain and dyspareunia (pain with sexual intercourse).

Pain, Dyspareunia, and Edema

While many obstetricians perceive it to be a minor problem, many women regard post-episiotomy pain as quite a serious matter.[28] The available medical literature supports the point of view that post-episiotomy pain can be severe for up to 60 percent of women undergoing the procedure.[4,7,26,36] Dyspareunia is also significant for about 20 percent of women for up to 3 months after delivery.[28] Edema is also frequent following episiotomy.[4,28]

Infection

Infection is another potentially serious complication of episiotomy that has not been looked at systematically. Stitch abscesses occur following episiotomy in approximately 1 percent of women; other types of wound infections and abscesses have been observed to occur in 0.5-3 percent of post-episiotomy patients.[21,29] There are three studies of particular concern in which the causes of maternal mortality were examined. Infection of the episiotomy site was found to occasionally lead to a serious problem called necrotizing fasciitis. Death associated with this problem accounted for 20-30 percent of all maternal mortality in the populations studied.[23,25,40] Because these reports are geographically based, the scope of this problem is unclear, but these papers certainly suggest that this rare but serious complication of episiotomy should be viewed with great concern.

SUMMARY

In conclusion, episiotomies are done frequently in the United States despite the absence of data to support such routine use. Moreover, there are significant risks associated with episiotomies that have not been adequately studied. What, then, is an optimal episiotomy rate for the United States? In birthing centers where nurse-midwives have primary responsibility, the episiotomy rate runs between 15-25 percent, with rates of third-degree lacerations of 3-4 percent and rates for first- and second-degree lacerations requiring repair of 25-30 percent.[19,24] In the absence of better data, our judgment is that the U.S. episiotomy rate could be reduced by more than half without causing harm to either mothers or babies. Systematic study of the benefits and risks associated with this procedure would provide an even better estimate of the optimal episiotomy rate and the circumstances in which that procedure is most clearly indicated.

REFERENCES

1. Aldridge AH, Watson P. Analysis of end-results of labor in primiparas after spontaneous versus prophylactic methods of delivery. J Obstet Gynecol 30:554-565, 1935.

2. Banta HD, Thacker SB. Assessing the costs and benefits of electronic fetal monitoring. Obstet Gynecol Surv 35:627-642, 1979.

3. Banta HD, Thacker SB. Electronic fetal monitoring: is it of benefit? Birth Fam J 6:237-249, 1979.

4. Bare WW, Fine ES. Prophylaxis of episiotomy pain: a controlled study of oral trypsins on the postpartum course. Am J Obstet Gynecol 87:268-271, 1963.

5. Beynon CL. The normal second stage of labour. J Obstet Gynaecol Br Commonw 64:815-820, 1957. (Reprinted in this volume.)

6. Bloomfield SS, Hurwitz HN. Tourniquet and episiotomy pain as test models for aspirin-like analgesics. J Clin Pharmacol 10:361-369, 1970.

7. Boutselis JG, Sollars RJ. The effect of proteolytic enzymes on episiotomy pain and swelling. Ohio State Med J 60:551-553, 1964.

8. Bowes WA. Obstetrical Medication and Infant Outcome: A Review of the Literature. The Effects of Obstetrical Medication on Fetus and Infant. Monographs of the Society for Research in Child Development, Serial #137; 35:3-23, 1970.

9. Brendsel C, Peterson G, Mehl LE. Episiotomy: facts, fictions, figures, and alternatives. In: Stewart D and Stewart L, eds. Compulsory Hospitalization or Freedom of Choice in Childbirth? Marble Hill, MO: National Association

of Parents and Professionals for Safe Alternatives in Childbirth (NAPSAC), 1979.

10. Buchan PC, Nicholls JAJ. Pain after episiotomy--a comparison of two methods of repair. J Roy Col Gen Pract 30:297-300, 1980.

11. Bureau of the Census: Historical Statistics of the United States, Colonial Times to 1970. Washington, D.C. Vol. 53, 1975.

12. Bureau of the Census: Fertility of American Women. Current Population Reports 1980. Series P-20-350, June 1979.

13. Caldeyro-Barcia R. The influence of maternal bearing-down efforts during second stage on fetal well-being. Birth Fam J 6:17-21, 1979. (Reprinted in this volume.)

14. Caldeyro-Barcia R. Personal communication, 1981.

15. Chalmers I, Richards M. Intervention and causal inference in obstetric practice. In: Chard T, Richards M, eds. Benefits and Hazards of the New Obstetrics. Lavenham, Suffolk: The Lavenham Press, Ltd., 1977, pp.34-61.

16. Child CG. Episiotomy: its relation to the proper conduct of the perineal stage of labor. Med Rec 96:142-144, 1919.

17. Coats PM, Chan KK, Wilkins M, et al. A comparison between midline and mediolateral episiotomies. Br J Obstet Gynaecol 87:408-412, 1980.

18. Cogan R, Edmonds EP. The unkindest cut? J Nurs Midw 23:17-21, 1978.

19. Cranch J. Personal communication, 1981.

20. DeLee JB. The prophylactic forceps operation. Am J Obstet Gynecol 1:34-44, 1920.

21. Diethelm MW. Episiotomy: technique of repair. Ohio State Med J 34:1107-1111, 1938.

22. Douglas RG, Stromme WB. Operative obstetrics. In: Management of Delivery Trauma. Third Edition. New York: Appleton-Century-Crofts, 1976.

23. Ewing TL, Smale LE, Elliott FA. Maternal deaths associated with postpartum vulvar edema. Am J Obstet Gynecol 134:173-179, 1979.

24. Gaskin IM. Community alternatives to high technology birth. In: Holmes HB, Hoskins BB, Gross M, eds. Birth Control and Controlling Birth. Humana Press Inc., Clifton, New Jersey, 1980, pp. 223-229.

25. Golde S, Ledger WJ. Necrotizing fasciitis in postpartum patients. Obstet Gynecol 50:670-673, 1977.

26. Huff GD. Mediolateral episiotomy. Calif West Med 48:177-179, 1938.

27. Kantor HI, Rember R, Tabio P, et al. Value of shaving the pudendal-perineal area in delivery preparation. Obstet Gynecol 25:509-512, 1965.

28. Kitzinger S, Walters R. Some Women's Experience of Episiotomy. National Childbirth Trust, London, 1981.

29. Kretzschmar NR, Huber CP. A study of 2987 consecutive episiotomies. Am J Obstet Gynecol 35:621-626, 1938.

30. Mandy TE, Christhilf SM, Mandy AJ, et al. Evaluation of the Rucker method of episiotomy repair as to perineal pain. Am J Surg 82:251-255, 1951.

31. Marieskind H. An Evaluation of Cesarean Section in the United States Washington D.C.: Department of Health, Education, and Welfare, June 1979.

32. Mehl LE. The outcome of home delivery research in the United States. In: Kitzinger S, Davis JA, eds. The Place of Birth. Oxford University Press, New York, 1979, pp. 91-117.

33. National Center for Health Statistics. Data from the Hospital Discharge Survey. Furnished by Eileen McCarthy, 1981.

34. National Institutes of Health, National Institute of Child Health and Human Development. Antenatal Diagnosis, Report of a Consensus Development Conference. NIH Publication No. 79-1973. Bethesda, Md., 1979.

35. Nelson KB, Broman SH. Perinatal risk factors in children with serious motor and mental handicaps. Ann Neurol 1977, 371-377.

36. Niswander K, Gordon M, Drage J. The effect of intrauterine hypoxia in the child surviving to 4 years. Am J Obstet Gynecol 121:892-899, 1975.

37. Nugent FB. The primiparious perineum after forceps delivery. Am J Obstet Gynecol 30:249-256, 1935.

38. Pomeroy RH. Shall we cut and reconstruct the perineum for every primipara? Am J Obstet Dis Wom Child 78:211-220, 1918.

39. Pritchard JA, MacDonald PC. Williams Obstetrics. 16th Edition. New York: Appleton-Century-Crofts, 1980.

40. Shy KK, Eschenbach DA. Fatal perineal cellulitis from an episiotomy site. Obstet Gynecol 54:292-298, 1979.

41. Thacker SB, Banta HD. Benefits and risks of episiotomy. Women and Health 7:161-177, 1982.

42. Thacker SB, Banta HD. Benefits and risks of episiotomy, an interpretative review of the English-language literature, 1860-1980. Obstet Gynecol Surv 38(6):322-338, Nov 83.

43. Wertz RW, Wertz DC. Lying-in, A History of Childbirth in America. New York: The Plenum Press, 1977.

44. Wood C, Ng KH, Hounslow D, et al. Time--an important variable in normal delivery. J Obstet Gynaecol Br Commonw 80:295-300, 1973.

10. To Do or Not To Do Episiotomy?

M.J. House, M.R.C.O.G.

Though there is extensive literature discussing the angle of cut, the craft of suturing and the type of suture material which should be used, there is little questioning of the need for the episiotomy to be done in the first place or suggesting how it might be avoided. The practice of episiotomy has been so thoroughly incorporated into the Western way of birth that it has become an anticipated and normal part of childbirth for most women, and is often not even perceived as an intervention. In this chapter a consultant obstetrician queries the widespread use of episiotomy.

HISTORICAL BACKGROUND

Episiotomy has been an established practice since the early part of this century and it is now practiced in the so-called civilized world with an instance of between 30 and 70 percent of all deliveries. The various methods of performing this operation and of managing the side effects have all been well documented but it must be stressed at the outset that there is an almost complete lack of any scientific evidence that the operation has any of the beneficial effects claimed for it. A search of the literature has failed to reveal any study designed to compare the effects on mother and baby of doing or not doing episiotomies.

INDICATIONS

The indications for doing episiotomies are unfortunately so well known and well documented that they are accepted by student, midwife and doctor alike without question. However, in brief, they are to protect the mother's perineum and to facilitate delivery of the baby in various circumstances.

A careful look at these indications, however, reveals that there is little real evidence that either of these things is achieved. The operation itself cuts across natural skin folds and across muscles and any surgeon of experience knows that these factors are associated with relatively poor healing.

Poor and/or delayed healing is of course associated with pain and in my experience, it is not uncommon to see a patient, following an uncomplicated cesarean section with a Pfannenstiel incision move around the ward more easily and with more confidence than a patient who has had an uncomplicated so-called normal delivery but with the 'benefit' of the almost inevitable episiotomy.

We as obstetricians teach that episiotomy prevents tears and reduces the likelihood of prolapse in the future but we have little or no evidence for making these statements. Not only is there no evidence that episiotomy prevents tears but there is some evidence to the contrary.[5]

In a recent article by Mr. J.S. Fox [5] there are some very interesting figures. In 1971, at his hospital, patients delivered in the so-called Domino Scheme had an episiotomy rate of four per cent and tear rate of 15 per cent. [Editor's note: Domino is a scheme whereby community midwives go with their patients into hospital during labor, deliver them there and then bring them home again a few hours after.] By 1977, that episiotomy rate, for a variety of reasons had risen to 38 per cent and the tear rate at that time had also risen to 23 per cent.

Without further details, it would be impossible to say that the rise in tears was significant, but certainly, there was no indication at all that the dramatic rise in the number of episiotomies done was in any way associated with a reduction in the number of tears. It is also most unlikely that midwives were getting much worse performing normal deliveries during these years, but there is no doubt that the dramatic rise in the episiotomy rate was associated with the fact that doctors became more and more available to repair the episiotomies done. Harris[6], in reviewing this situation, reported a 22 per cent tear rate in primiparous women who had an episiotomy.

At a recent meeting I attended on the subject of episiotomies, it was fairly seriously suggested that it was far easier to teach people (in this case medical students), episiotomy and repair than it was to teach a properly conducted controlled delivery with an acceptable tear rate.

What of tears themselves? Are they as serious as we have been led to believe? Again there is no evidence that they need occur with anything like the frequency that episiotomy is performed [3,4] or that when they do, they are in any way more painful, heal more slowly or give rise to more long term problems.

A number of authors [7, 11, 12] have suggested that damage to the pelvic floor commonly occurs even in the absence of visible tears, but except in the case of forceps delivery, the evidence is lacking.[10]

It would seem then, that there is little evidence to support the operation to protect the mother. However, any experienced obstetrician knows that there are a number of circumstances in which it is necessary.

Forceps delivery with the possible exception of a late Wrigley's lift-out, cannot be done without episiotomy or almost certainly a bad tear will result. In the case of breech delivery and a premature labor, especially in primigravid patients I feel it is also essential, although even in this case, I feel each case must be judged on its merits at the time. In these days of defensive medicine, we should not allow fear of the occasional tear to pressure midwives and obstetricians alike into doing elective episiotomy on the vast majority of patients.

THE TECHNIQUE

The technique of midline and medio-lateral episiotomies is already well documented and the multitude of articles on alternate suture materials and methods of repair suggests that no one is perfect.

Controversies still exist between the standard medio-lateral episiotomy and the midline, but the available evidence would suggest that the dangers of the midline episiotomy have been exaggerated.

It is therefore not my intentions to go over old ground but to raise a number of questions that I feel need answering. Firstly, do all birth attendants know when an episiotomy should be done? My observations lead me to believe that they do not and the more inexperienced the attendant, the earlier the episiotomy would seem to be done.

I believe it is quite barbarous to do an episiotomy without a local anesthetic except in dire emergency, but hidden in this old practice there is some good. The timing was right. The cut should be delayed until the perineal tissues are well stretched and there are many reasons for this:

1. Before this time it is not possible to judge whether or not episiotomy will be necessary. However, if the suspicion is there and the patient does not have an epidural, the region may be infiltrated with local anesthetic and the right time awaited.

2. Cutting the perineum before it distends is quite pointless as it does not hasten completion of the second stage. Episiotomies are often done too early in the second stage because the presenting part is visible but descending rather slowly. However, if the perineum is not stretched by the head, then the lack of progress in the second stage is due to something else and an episiotomy will help no one.

3. Blood loss: The volume of blood loss at episiotomy is nearly always grossly underestimated and one only has to check the hemoglobins of patients in the postnatal ward with recorded blood losses of between 200 and 300 ml to confirm this. Too early an episiotomy I believe, often leads to undetected and certainly unrecorded blood loss in excess of 500 ml and this loss is often compounded by delay in completing the repair.

4. Technical problems: Too early an episiotomy is technically more difficult than cutting the perineum when it is well stretched. Tissues may well move away from the

scissors blades especially if they are not the sharpest, leading to either repeated attempts at cut and a ragged edge or what is probably worse, to an inadequate incision.

Too small an incision may well lead to an extension of the episiotomy with a tear which goes down towards the rectum and this makes for a very difficult repair job.

At this point, I would like to enter a plea for immediate repair of episiotomy. One of the worst experiences of the mothers in childbirth is to be 'left for ages' before the repair is done. Most mothers, as is the case with patients having major surgery think that 'the stitches' are the worst part of the whole affair and it is important that we bear these words in mind. It is 'the stitches' not the cutting that are uppermost in a patient's mind.

If for any reason, the birth attendant is not the one who will be doing the repair, then he or she must be there in time to carry straight on after the delivery. Any number of rituals are often attended to instead of getting on with the repair but the only factor that should allow delay of any kind to take place is a very ill baby, or possibly some other complication in the mother.

This brings me to the question of who should be doing episiotomy and who should repair it. In order to get a satisfactory result, the repair of an episiotomy often requires more skill than a routine appendectomy and the aftereffects of a bad job are far more apparent to the patient and cause endless physical and psychological distress. For many reasons, I feel that it is in the best interests of the patient that the person doing the episiotomy should also repair it. Midwives, therefore, should be well trained in both the procedure and its repair and it should never be left to someone of limited experience. The temptation to regard the episiotomy repair as a minor procedure after the major event of delivery is safely over must be resisted.

Inexperience leads to misalignment of tissues, over-tightening of sutures. The latter may cause some ischemia which may then lead to pain, infection and/or breakdown of repair. We all know, especially, when the initial relief and delight of a normal childbirth are over, the endless misery that can be caused by a painful perineum.

RESULTS

It would be expected that for a standard procedure, that is performed hundreds of thousands of times every year there would be solid evidence in the world literature comparing the results of delivery with and without episiotomy. Without such evidence, how could such a widespread procedure become so well established? In fact, no such evidence exists. As already mentioned, there are some fairly ancient reports comparing the results on the perineum of delivery by forceps with and without episiotomy but no such comparison has been made with normal deliveries.

Since therefore, there is no direct evidence of benefit, what of the side effects?

1. Pain: This is what concerns a patient most immediately postpartum. She has been through a long, trying and painful day and there is often a certain sense of anticlimax after the delivery is complete. If she then has to have an episiotomy, she may then have a painful tail, although this can be minimized by careful repair. There are endless articles of the various methods of pain relief and drugs that can be used following episiotomies but any woman who has had one could give evidence that prevention is certainly better than the cure.

By prevention, I mean firstly reducing the incidence of episiotomy overall and secondly careful and expert repair in all cases. The well repaired episiotomy even if an extension has occurred should not be very painful.

2. Bleeding: This I have already discussed and there is plenty of evidence to suggest that blood loss due to episiotomy is almost always underestimated. [8,12]

3. Breakdown: This is unfortunately not an uncommon event and its incidence is inversely related to the experience and expertise of the person doing the repair. Minor degrees of breakdown cause a delayed healing but a complete breakdown will require re-suturing. This inevitably results in a messy wound after a protracted stay in hospital. Re-suturing of a broken episiotomy is notoriously difficult and the end result is rarely entirely satisfactory.

In my experience, tears rarely break down, but again, there seems to be no evidence comparing the results of repair of episiotomies with repair of tears. It could be that bad tears are repaired by someone of more experience and therefore a better job is done, but I feel it is more likely that the blood supply to the edges of the tear are better than is the case with episiotomy.

4. Long term problems: Fortunately, even after the worst episiotomy, with extensions, breakdowns, etc., in the due course of time, (which may be weeks or even months in rare cases), the final result is usually fairly satisfactory and symptoms eventually do fade away.

However, in a small minority of patients, dyspareunia persists and this is usually quite unrelated to any detectable anatomical defect. Beischer [1] in a long term follow-up of episiotomy found that dyspareunia persisted in six percent of patients. I find this rather a high figure but it may well be that in hospital practice, we do not see quite a lot of the long term problems that we cause. Furthermore, there is no evidence that restoration of anatomical 'normality' leads to functional normality or increased sexual satisfaction.

There seems to be nothing in the literature about the long term follow-up of patients without episiotomy, with and without tears, but my feeling is that similar problems do not occur in this group to anything like the same extent.

CONCLUSION

Episiotomy is now a well established part of obstetric care all over the world where medical attention is readily available. It is performed in the interests of mother and child with all the good intentions in the world but with little evidence that in fact it benefits either.

However, it has a number of well established undesirable side effects and this has resulted in a huge volume of literature on the various ways to minimize these problems.

This chapter is written in order to enter a plea of a complete reappraisal of the whole situation and in hope that a drastic reduction in the incidence of this 'minor' operation can be achieved in the future.

REFERENCES

1. BEISCHER N.A. The anatomical and functional results of mediolateral episiotomy, Med J Aust 2:189, 1967.

2. BEYNON C.L. Midline episiotomy as a routine procedure J Obstet Gynaecol Br Commonw 81:126, 1974.

3. CLARKE A.P. The management of the perineum during labour. Trans Am Assoc Obstet Gynecol 2:206, 1889.

4. DEWEES W.B. Relaxation and management of the perineum during parturition. JAMA 13:804, 1889.

5. FOX J.S. Episiotomy. Midwives Chronical & Nursing Notes 337-340, 1979.

6. HARRIS R.E. An evaluation of the median episiotomy. Am J Obstet Gynecol 106:660, 1970.

7. INMON W.B. Mediolaterial episiotomy. South Med J 53:257, 1960.

8. NEWTON M., MOSEY L.M., EGLI G.E., et al. Blood loss during and immediately after delivery. Obstet Gynecol 17-9, 1961.

9. NOBLE E. Clinical evaluation of the pelvic floor. Paper presented at the International Childbirth Education Association Convention Kansas City, 1978.

10. NUGENT F.B. The primiparous perineum after forceps delivery. A follow-up comparison of results with and without episiotomy. Am J Obstet Gynecol 30:249, 1935.

11. SHUTE, W.B. A physiologic appraisal and a new painless technic. Obstet Gynecol 14:467, 1959.

12. TRITSCH J.E. Another plea for the prophylatic median episiotomy. Am Inst Homeopath 23:327, 1930.

11. The Midline Episiotomy.

Yehudi Gordon, M.D., M.R.C.O.G., F.C.O.G. (S.A.)

Episiotomy and suturing of the perineum can be traumatic for the mother, and for many women the post-partum experience is marred by severe perineal discomfort. Some say that episiotomy and suturing of the perineum was more painful than anything in labor itself and it is the thing they dread most about having another baby. Postpartum pain may interfere with the mother's early relationship with her baby and the establishing of breast-feeding. In this chapter a consultant who favors the midline position as occurring in a site where healing takes place more easily, describes how it should be done and the correct method of suturing the perineum.

INTRODUCTION

Episiotomy is the commonest invasive procedure performed during the lifetime of any woman. The other events which occur during childbirth tend to focus the woman's attention away from her incised vagina and perineum but in the absence of these other stimuli it is likely that the long-term psychological effects of episiotomy would be increased. If the outcome of the pregnancy is successful, the woman has a new baby to act as a focus of attention and the pain and discomfort resulting from the episiotomy is accepted. A number of general points relating to the complications should be considered.

The long term psychological sequelae of episiotomy can be reduced if the following principles are adhered to. First, the minimum amount of tissue damage should be present. Second, the rate of healing and pain associated with healing should be optimal. Third, the mother should be given a clear explanation during delivery and again during the postnatal period about the reasons for undertaking the procedure.

ANATOMICAL CONSIDERATIONS

The superficial and deep pelvic muscles surrounding the vagina meet in the midline anteriorly and posteriorly. At the junction there are no muscle fibres and a central tendon is present between the vagina and anus (Figure 1). It is obvious that a midline episiotomy has a number of major advantages. (Figure 2). First, the incision is through the connective tissue and not through muscle fibres. Second, the incision is as far as possible from the major blood vessels to the pelvis. The vessels enter from the lateral side wall veins and arteries is small. Third, the anatomical forces tend to maintain the cut ends in apposition after delivery.

By contrast, a mediolateral episiotomy has many disadvantages (Figure 2). The incision involves cutting across muscle fibres and blood vessels. This leads to an increased loss of blood and the stimulated muscle fibres contract thus widening and distorting the original incision. The distortion leads to technical problems of accurate apposition of the cut edges during the repair. During the post-operative period the stimulated fibres are likely to undergo spasm thus creating pain by tension on the sutures as well as distortion of the incision and scar tissue formation. The cut vessels also lead to an increase in pressure in the pelvic veins and may result in hemorrhoids formation or breakdown of the wound because of hematoma formation.

MIDLINE VERSUS MEDIOLATERAL EPISIOTOMY

	Midline	Mediolateral
1. Repair:	Easy	Difficulty increases with the size of the incision
2. Blood Loss:	Less	Greater
3. Puerperal pain:	Rare	Universal
4. Associated Hemorrhoids	Less	Greater
5. Anatomical apposition:	Usually good	Commonly faulty
6. Dyspareunia and scar tenderness:	Rare	Not uncommon
7. Third degree extension:	Not uncommon	Rare

The only disadvantage of a midline episiotomy is extension of the incision backwards into the perianal muscles, anus and rectum, causing a third degree tear. If this is recognized and repaired immediately the results are usually excellent. There is, however, a small risk of development of a recto-vaginal fistula which will require subsequent admission to hospital and repair under general anesthesia.

HOW TO AVOID A THIRD DEGREE TEAR

The most important factor in avoiding extension of the midline episiotomy into the rectum is gentle delivery of the head of the baby and particularly of the posterior shoulder. The anus should be supported with a gauze swab.

There are a number of circumstances in which a midline episiotomy is contraindicated and a mediolateral episiotomy is preferable. These include women with a short perineum, delivery of the aftercoming head of a breech or where forceps are being used to rotate the head from a posterior to an anterior position.

REPAIR OF A MIDLINE EPISIOTOMY

The repair is begun at the apex of the vaginal incision using a continuous 00 atraumatic catgut suture. This suture should be tied just inside the hymen (Figure 3). Next three of four interrupted catgut sutures are placed in the cut central tendon to appose the superficial and deep perineal muscles. Excessive tension should be avoided (Figure 4). The subcutaneous fascia is now united using a continuous suture which begins immediately below the fourchette and ends at the posterior margin of the episiotomy (Figure 5). This continuous suture is now carried upward as a subcuticular stitch to obtain apposition of the skin edges. The area between the hymen and the fourchette is not sutured to prevent subsequent dyspareunia.

REPAIR OF A THIRD DEGREE TEAR

The rectal mucosa is sutured with interrupted catgut sutures, with the knots tied away from the rectal lumen. The severed sphincter is identified and resutured with two or three interrupted catgut sutures (Figure 6). The midline episiotomy is now sutured.

EPISIOTOMY CARE DURING THE PUERPERIUM

Even after a third degree tear no special care is needed during the puerperium. The mother is encouraged to bathe the area twice a day and to avoid nylon underwear. When pain is present, analgesic tablets are helpful and hemorrhoids usually respond to suppositories administered locally.

PELVIC PAIN FOLLOWING EPISIOTOMY

Even after the most carefully performed and sutured episiotomy, pain in the suture line or in the middle or upper vagina is a not uncommon occurrence. Fortunately, in the post-natal period this pain tends to settle spontaneously and only a small percentage of women will be left with long-term discomfort. It is essential at this stage to differentiate between pain in the suture line and general levator ani muscle dysfunction. In the former case a vaginal examination will show local tenderness over the suture line with almost no tenderness in the surrounding musculature. It is frequent, however, to find that the sacrum is tilted following delivery and this causes pain radiating from the sacroiliac joint and along the levator ani muscles. If the tilt is to the right and the episiotomy is also to the right, tension on the right levator ani muscle will cause an increased amount of pain in the area of the episiotomy. This complication can be fairly easily dealt with by manipulation of the sacrum in the post-natal period. It is often very useful for the woman to be informed about the cause of the discomfort and to be assured that resumption of normal sexual intercourse will actually improve matters.

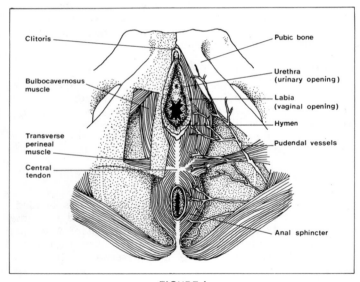

FIGURE I

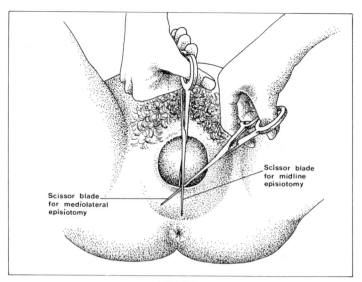

Scissor blade
for mediolateral
episiotomy

Scissor blade
for midline
episiotomy

FIGURE 2

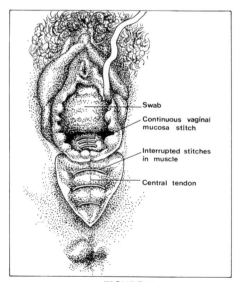

Swab

Continuous vaginal
mucosa stitch

Interrupted stitches
in muscle

Central tendon

FIGURE 3

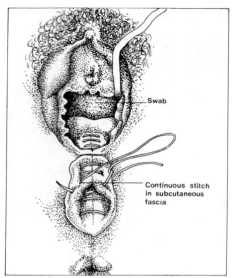

FIGURE 4

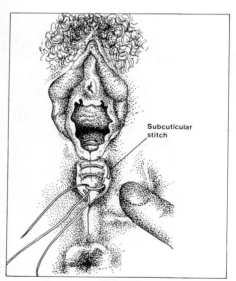

FIGURE 5

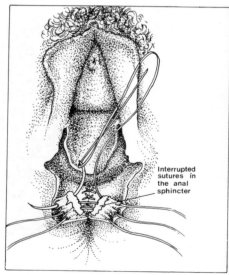

FIGURE 6

12. Episiotomy, Body Image and Sex

Sheila Kitzinger, M.Litt.

Episiotomy turns birth, however natural it is otherwise, into a surgical operation. Invasion of tissue always produces some trauma and the woman needs time to recover from the wound. For a newly delivered mother this time corresponds with that during which she is beginning to learn how to interact with her baby and trying to establish breastfeeding. There is another relationship which is almost invariably affected, to a greater or lesser degree -- that with the sexual partner. Episiotomy is surgical incision of the sexual organs, so it is not surprising that many women experience dyspareunia for weeks or months afterwards. This chapter looks at the effects which episiotomy may have on self-image and the relationship between the sexual partners, and discusses the emotionally supportive counselling which can assist postnatal sexual adjustment.

After childbirth a woman's feelings about her body and the way in which she pictures her sexual organs are mingled with all the psycho-physical experience of what should be recognized as a fourth trimester of pregnancy. Dramatic changes are occurring over a short space of time. The woman was full. She is now empty. Her abdomen was firm and rounded. Now it is flat -- but flabby as a collapsed cream puff. Her breasts are throbbing and swollen, criss-crossed with veins like rivers and their tributaries. Her nipples are dark, erect and prominent. Before the birth her body was closed. Now it is open. And in the early postpartum weeks it is leaking blood, clots, mucus, perhaps urine, too. Moisture oozes from the whole skin surface and she may feel in a permanent bath of sweat. Her breasts leak colostrum and, later, milk. Her body is raw, vulnerable and exposed to the gaze and handling of others.

Any woman may feel like this during those first postpartum days and weeks. One who has had an episiotomy, especially if her permission was not asked beforehand, may also feel violated. That is a word many women use when talking about their reaction to episiotomy.

Episiotomy can be a minor cut which quickly heals. It is for many women, however, a wound which leaves them feeling scarred. The study I did on episiotomy for the National Childbirth Trust (N.C.T.)[1] revealed that by the end of the first week after delivery there was a highly significant difference not only between women who had been sutured and those who had not, but between those who had episiotomies and those with lacerations (Table 1). Women who had torn were much more likely to be comfortable than those who had episiotomies.

TABLE I

Comfort of perineum at end of 1st week (excluding cesarean births and forceps deliveries) in percentages (n=1129).

	Comfortable or mildly uncomfortable	Painful or very painful	No information	Total
Tear	84	15	1	100
Episiotomy and episiotomy + tear	62	37	1	100
Intact perineum	93	2	5	100

Eleven percent of women in this study were told they had an infection, which was treated with antibiotics. One women said: "At my postnatal checkup my GP told me that the stitches were not healing properly. He sent me back to the hospital where I was an outpatient for nearly four months, because I had to be cut and restitched and had to have an infection treated. Tests showed that both my fallopian tubes are blocked, resulting, the consultant has told me, from the infection contracted after my episiotomy."

Another said: "Four out of five of us who were friends came away from the hospital with an infection. I was sent home after seven days with stitches the hospital knew were breaking down but neither my midwife or doctor were informed. My doctor examined me and said I would have to go back and be restitched. However when I returned to the hospital they said I was too infected to be restitched and gave me antibiotics. Eventually, nine weeks after the baby was born, the infection cleared up."

But even when there is no sepsis women often say that they feel they are "sitting on thorns." Such acute pain in an already tender area may affect the way a woman holds and handles her baby and interfere with the easy start of breastfeeding. The N.C.T. study showed that women who have torn are more likely to be able to hold their babies comfortably than those who have had episiotomies. Fifty-five percent of those with lacerations could sit easily when holding the baby at the end of the first week, but only 27% of those who had episiotomies.

When pain of this kind persists it is bound to affect a couple's sexual relationship, and, because episiotomy tends to have emotional as well as physical effects, this may be the case even when the woman is expertly sutured and healing is rapid. Many women in the N.C.T. study experienced prolonged dyspareunia. Those who had episiotomies were much

more likely to find intercourse painful for more than one
month than those who had lacerations. One woman wrote:
"After three months I found that to have intercourse hurt
and afterwards I was very sore. One day I used a mirror to
look at myself down there and I saw a ridge of skin hanging
down a kind of split. I went to my doctor and he said the
stitches must come out and the split heal up . . . .
sometimes when we have intercourse my husband thinks he has
entered me, but his penis has gone against the tear, gone in
a little, then it closes and this hurts me very much."

Another wrote: "Lovemaking was impossible because of
excruciating pain; when he withdrew there was blood
trickling." She said that she was operated on to remove scar
tissue at 8 months post partum but looking back at what she
had been through commented: "It's been a very miserable and
depressing time. It certainly puts me off having another
baby." Another woman, who is herself a midwife, wrote: "From
my own experience I can tell you that episiotomies can be
agonizing. It is still sore to make love (one year after the
birth), so the spontaneity of it has gone. We always have to
make love rather carefully." Yet another woman said: "After
this awful experience with an episiotomy, plus an infection
on the stitches, plus postnatal depression and a 'difficult'
baby, and no intercourse because of the painful scar, I felt
that I never wanted another child ever."

With the first attempts at intercourse after childbirth
a pattern of anxiety and of acute pain can be laid down
which may persist long past the time when there is any
obvious physical reason for discomfort. Lying in the same
position for intercourse as that in which she was sutured
may trigger anxiety, anger and revulsion. It is often
difficult for a man to realize this. It means that the style
of lovemaking and the usual coital postures need to be
adapted and that the couple need to talk together about
their feelings. Then the sexual partner is helped to become
empathetically aware of how the woman is feeling and ready
to modify sexual techniques in order to meet her needs.

The doctor who operates on and subsequently sutures the
perineum often treats this exquisitely sensitive part of a
woman's sexual organs as an inanimate object. It might as
well be a football to be mended. He is faced with a
mechanical problem that needs putting right. This attitude
is forcefully conveyed to the woman. It is almost as if her
vagina and perineum are no longer part of herself. The
process of suturing and the pain felt at the time and
afterwards tend to alienate her from this part of her body.
She often does not want to look at the stitching in a mirror
or to touch it. She is aware only of pain and is frightened
of what she might find if she examined herself. Under these
circumstances any sexual approaches from her partner, any
suggestion that she might find pleasure in this area of her

body, can be anxiety-arousing. An invading penis — even a finger — may cause an involuntary muscle spasm. She feels attacked.

A woman who has been sutured too tightly, not allowing for the swelling of the tissue which follows injury, or who has been sutured by a medical student determined to do a thorough job, and stitching over and over again with intricate embroidery, feels that it would be impossible ever to have intercourse again. This is especially the case if she has received the extra "husband's stitch" which some American obstetricians take pride in doing. The woman's vagina is physically returned to a virgin state and sometimes almost to a pre-pubescent size.

Counselling after episiotomy, particularly sexual counselling, must always take into account both the physical and the emotional effects of having been cut and sutured. Immediate postpartum perineal pain is often helped by wearing a witch-hazel-soaked pad against the tender area, by sitz baths containing a handful of kitchen salt, and by gently stroking in a few drops of oil of arnica. Both warm air and cold compresses may help. The perineum can be exposed to the heat from a hand-held hair dryer or even an electric lamp. Alternatively, ice cubes wrapped in muslin or a diaper may also be comforting and assist healing by encouraging circulation in the area. Mobilization of the pelvic floor muscles, though difficult and painful at first, can gradually help fresh oxygenated blood to flow into the bruised tissues. Quite apart from the physical effects of exercise, doing pelvic floor movements can help the woman to get to know again and come to terms with her body after childbirth.

It may seem odd to insist that a woman needs to get to know her body again; after all, it has been hers all along. But emotional acceptance can be difficult when there has been a loss of part of the body (and this is how a woman has often felt about the fetus, as part of herself) -- the gaping hole where there was once a tooth, certainly an amputated limb, and the genitals after a woman has passed through the dramatic experience of birth.

Many women feel unable to explore their own vagina and perineum because they are afraid of what they will find. The small knot of scar tissue becomes magnified in their minds to the size of a large walnut. One way of helping a woman literally get in touch with her body again is by encouraging her to look at her perineum in a mirror, explore the area with her fingers and, gently and tentatively at first, to get her pelvic floor muscles flexible and moving.

Though intercourse is usually taken as the index of recovery in postnatal sexual adjustment it is important to stress that there are many ways of making love which do not involve penetration. After childbirth a couple might take

-106-

time to try other forms of lovemaking, not merely as a
preparation for intercourse, but because the woman needs to
be helped to feel good about her body -- her whole body. Men
often concentrate attention on sexual organs, especially the
clitoris, because they believe these are the source of
arousal. For many -- perhaps most -- women this is only half
true.[2] In a relationship with a sexual partner a woman is
likely to respond completely only when she feels desired as
a person and that every part of her body is beautiful.
Because episiotomy and suturing are sexually threatening
this is vital in the year after childbirth.

A good deal of publicity has been given to the clitoris
as the source of sexual arousal in a woman. The mistake made
by many men is to concentrate on the visible portion of this
organ and to rub it energetically. They often think that the
clitoris is like a miniature penis and will respond to the
same kind of stimulus. Masters and Johnson have a comment to
make on this: "Probably the greatest error that any man
makes approaching a woman sexually is that of direct attack
on the clitoral glans . . . ."[3] The tip of the clitoris is
in many women far too sensitive to tolerate heavy
stimulation. The man may not be aware that the larger part
of the clitoris, the root, is hidden. Slow stroking, sucking
or pressure against this area is usually more effective than
rubbing its tip as if he were Aladdin rubbing the lamp in
the expectation of instant ecstasy.

After episiotomy the woman may prefer her man to
ejaculate outside her. Semen spilled on the tender knot of
tissue increases comfort for some women and seems to help
tissues become more flexible. Other women dislike this and
find it messy.

If a couple want to have intercourse they may find it
helps to use pillows or a large floor cushion to tilt the
woman's pelvis, or the man's, so that there is no pressure
against the sutured area. This is often felt as a "knob" and
one advantage of looking at and exploring the area is that a
woman knows exactly where it is and can work out ways of
avoiding pressure against it during lovemaking.

A gel or oil smoothed into the tender tissues very
gently by the partner can merge with light, fingertip touch
of the root of the clitoris and the inner labia, a touch
which can become further as, and if, a woman enjoys it. She
may like to stroke oil on his penis, too.

Postures comfortable for intercourse are likely to be
those in which the woman has unhampered pelvic movement and
in which there is no heavy weight on tender, lactating
breasts. Some women find the "spoons" position a good one,
with the man lying behind the woman and her knees drawn up
and head and shoulders curved forward. Positions in which
penetration occurs from behind enable a woman to control the
degree of entry with contracted glutei. A female-superior

position may also make for more comfortable intercourse, since the woman can control the angle and depth of penetration in this way too.

Most episiotomy pain is experienced at the base of the vagina and a short distance inside. Once a finger or a penis is past this point then there is no pain at all. When there is pain deep in the vaginal vault it suggests damage to transcervical ligaments. This may take longer to heal.

The vagina is not a passive canal, merely a sheath for a penis. It can be, as we have seen in Chapter Three on Pelvic Floor Awareness, an active organ making "sucking," "kissing" and "squeezing" movements. Once the tip of the penis is introduced a couple may choose to lie relaxed and still so that the woman has a chance to feel comfortable with the penis inside her, knowing that her partner is leaving the action up to her. Or she may choose to draw the penis in further with her pelvic floor muscles. In all lovemaking after childbirth it is important that it is her choice and her initiative.

REFERENCES

1. Kitzinger S with Walters R. Some Women's Experiences of Episiotomy. London: National Childbirth Trust, 1981.

2. Kitzinger S. Woman's Experience of Sex. New York: Putnam, 1983.

3. Masters W and Johnson V. Human Sexual Inadequacy. London: J and A Churchill Ltd., 1970.

13. Review of Research Findings, 1984-1985.

Penny Simkin, R.P.T.

Here is a review of research findings on episiotomy and second stage management which have been reported since the First Edition of this book went to press. While the amount of interest is gratifying, particularly among midwives and nurses, notably lacking are papers from the prestigious departments of obstetrics in North America. Because episiotomy practices in North America are different from those in Europe, and because of the strong influence these departments have on standards of care, it is very unfortunate they have shown so little research interest.

Since the first edition of this book was published in mid-1984, concerns about episiotomy and second stage management are still high in priority for pregnant women contemplating their upcoming birth experiences. Women's desires to preserve their perineums, as well as the recent research findings on the subject have motivated some sensitive and concerned caregivers to learn and try the techniques described herein.

By no means are all the answers available as yet. Bias, preference, and past medical training still determine most caregivers' practices. However, recent research provides further enlightenment on the efficacy of episiotomy and on maternal position and bearing-down efforts during second stage. We will briefly review these reports here.

EFFICACY OF EPISIOTOMY

Two recent trials from England and Ireland compared outcomes when episiotomy was frequently performed and when it was rarely performed. These trials, both of which were prospectively designed randomized trials, failed to confirm the advantages usually proclaimed for episiotomy.

The West Berkshire trial[1], which included 1000 women, found that if episiotomies were performed almost exclusively for fetal indications, (about 11% of the time), low Apgar scores and admissions to special care nurseries were no more frequent, severe trauma to the perineum was not significantly greater, perineal pain was no different at 10 days and 3 months post partum, than in a group where episiotomies were frequently performed (51%). Resumption of intercourse within the first month after birth was more frequent in the group with fewer episiotomies.

The Dublin study[2] included 181 women, half of whom received a routine episiotomy (100%), the other half, only if medically indicated (8%). Pain in the first four postpartum days was measured. Those with an intact perineum (21%) had the lowest pain scores. Pain in those with first and second degree tears was similar to those with episiotomies, although women with epidural anesthesia plus episiotomies had the highest pain scores of all. There were no third-degree tears. Other findings included no indications of prolonged second stage, fetal head trauma, or greater damage to the pelvic floor when episiotomy was avoided.

A third descriptive report(3) from Sweden compared pain and healing in 123 primigravidas who received episiotomies (86% mediolateral, 14% median) with 31 primigravidas with spontaneous lacerations (28 which involved the perineum and 3 which involved the sphincter).

At 5 to 6 days post partum, the episiotomy group had more wound infections, hematomas, wound swelling, and poorer wound healing than the spontaneous laceration group. Pain experienced by the mothers was more severe on sitting and exercising in the episiotomy group.

Episiotomy is claimed to preserve muscle strength in the perineum by preventing undue stretching. The question of perineal muscle strength in primiparas and its relation to perineal trauma during childbirth has recently been investigated(4). Findings indicated that the amount and type of perineal trauma (intact perineum after vaginal birth, second degree laceration, episiotomy, and forceps plus episiotomy) was not related to perineal muscle function one year post partum. Furthermore, two control groups were also compared: women who had had cesarean sections and nulliparous women. Their perineal function was not significantly better than those in the various vaginal delivery groups.

The authors did find a significant positive correlation, however, between perineal muscle function and the amount of regular exercise taken by the women, regardless of degree of perineal trauma. Thus, the theory that episiotomy preserves perineal muscle function was not supported. The same is true for the belief that an intact perineum results in overstretching of the perineum. Rather, the importance of regular exercise, whether pure perineal exercise or other potentially less "tedious" exercise, was confirmed in this study.

The reader should bear in mind that the usual incision in Ireland, the UK and Scandinavia is mediolateral, running across the perineal muscle, instead of midline, where it follows a natural line between muscles. The midline is the usual in the United States and is widely used in Canada. One study(5) suggests that midline episiotomies heal more readily than mediolateral episiotomies, and that intercourse is resumed earlier.

Therefore, we can only speculate on the applicability of these studies to North American women who have had midline episiotomies. The need is urgent for North American research on episiotomy.

THE SQUATTING POSITION FOR BIRTH

Two recent reports on outcomes associated with the squatting position for birth provide the first descriptive data on the utilization of that position by women unaccustomed to using squatting as opposed to chair-sitting as their usual resting position.

One report retrospectively compared maternal and fetal outcomes in two similar populations whose caregivers held similar non-interventive philosophies of maternity care(6). A major difference between the two study groups was that one group (n=200) used the squatting position for birth and the other (n=100) were semi-recumbent or sidelying. The squatting group fared better than the semi-recumbent group in several outcomes: for example, second stage was shorter in the squatting group (by 23 minutes in primigravidas and 13 minutes in multiparas); there were fewer mechanically assisted deliveries in primigravidas (7.5% vs 17.3%); fewer severe perineal lacerations (1% vs 14%); fewer episiotomies (7% vs 37%); and more intact perineums (45.5% vs 18%). Other differences were not significant.

In the other report(7), 30% of all 179 deliveries taking place during the study period were in the squatting position. Seventeen other women used the squatting position during second stage, but not for birth. Thirty-six per cent of those who squatted for birth had intact perineums; 29% had first degree lacerations; 29% had second degree lacerations; 7% had episiotomies. There was one third degree extension of an episiotomy.

Fetal and neonatal outcomes were not reported.

Although these studies were not prospective or adequately controlled for possible confounding variables, they indicate that the squatting position deserves serious consideration as an intervention to improve the course of second stage for both mother and infant. Other positions, as well as the principle of maternal choice of position, also deserve fair investigation.

One attempt to investigate associations between perineal outcomes and maternal delivery positions was inconclusive because of a lack of variety of birth positions in the populations studied. Eighty-three per cent of the 847 home births studied were in semi-sitting, reflecting the preferences of the seven physicians attending the births(8). Other positions utilized were distributed between hands and knees (7.6%), lateral Sim's (5.3%), squatting (1.6%), and lithotomy (0.1%).

The influence of maternal bearing-down efforts was examined in a small pilot study of 10 women(9). Half were taught sustained breath-holding and bearing down throughout second-stage contractions. The other half were taught only to follow their involuntary urge to bear down. During labor, they were reminded and encouraged to do as they had been taught.

The assumptions that prolonged bearing down and breathholding shortens second stage and results in higher Apgar scores were not confirmed. In fact, the findings suggest that involuntary bearing-down efforts are accompanied by adequate labor progress and result in less perineal trauma.

This study's findings, although hampered by the small sample size, are consistent with those reported by Caldeyro-Barcia and Beynon, in this volume.

CONCLUSION

All the recent studies reviewed here add strength to the arguments presented in this book, that the benefits of a non-interventive approach to second stage management may exceed those of a more aggressive approach. More carefully controlled studies are needed to test the beliefs which have dictated second stage management over the past half century.

Once a non-aggressive approach is deemed no more harmful than the aggressive approach, the next step will be to perfect this new approach to further improve outcomes, and decrease the number and severity of spontaneous lacerations. We need to find out the true benefit of the Kegel and other exercises, of prenatal perineal massage. Should a woman really do 100 pelvic floor contractions a day? What support measures, if any, preserve the integrity of the perineum -- hot compresses, massage with oil, pressure, proper coaching of the woman? What is the relationship between the mother's position and bearing-down efforts to fetal and maternal outcomes, both short- and long-term? Can one predict the circumstances under which episiotomy is beneficial? How do outcomes without episiotomy compare with outcomes with mediolateral and midline episiotomies?

Because long-lasting dyspareunia is a frequent complaint after childbirth, and seems related to perineal trauma, whether caused by laceration or episiotomy(10), it is urgent that we improve our ability to prevent such a distressing outcome of childbirth.

These and many other questions render the second stage of labor still a fertile area for research. In the meantime those who wish to perfect their skills in physiologic management will continue to benefit from the ideas and suggestions presented in this book.

REFERENCES

1. Sleep J, et al. West Berkshire perineal management trial. Br Med J 289(6445):587-590, 8 Sep 84.

2. Harrison RF, et al. Is routine episiotomy necessary? Br Med Jr 288(6435):1971-75, 30 Jun 84.

3. Rockner G, et al. A descriptive study of episiotomy and spontaneous laceration of perineum during childbirth. Paper presented before the International Confederation of Midwives, Sydney, Australia, Sep 84.

4. Gordon H and M Logue Perineal muscle function after childbirth. Lancet 2(8447):123-125, 20 Jul 85.

5. Coats PM, et al. A comparison between midline and mediolateral episiotomies. Br J Obstet Gynaecol 87:408-412, 1980.

6. Vedam S and J Golay. The squatting position for second stage of labor: Effects on the evolution and progress of labor and on maternal and fetal well-being. Master's Thesis, Yale University School of Nursing. May 85.

7. Kurokawa J and M Zilkoski. Adapting hospital obstetrics to birth in the squatting position. Birth 12(2):87-90, Summer 85.

8. Roberts JE and DM Kirz. Delivery positions and perineal outcome. J Nurs Midwif 29(3):186-90, May/Jun 84.

9. Yeates DA and JE Roberts. A comparison of two bearing-down techniques during the second stage of labor. J Nurs Midwif 29(1):3-11, Jan/Feb 84.

10. Ryding EL. Sexuality during and after pregnancy. Acta Obstet Gynecol Scand 63:679-682, 1984.

Appendix A. Prenatal Perineal Massage

Penny Simkin, R.P.T.

(Adapted from Pregnancy, Childbirth and the Newborn: A Complete Guide for Expectant Parents, by Penny Simkin, Janet Whalley and Ann Keppler. Deephaven MN, Meadowbrook Books, 1984.)

Perineal massage is used to soften the tissue around the vagina and increase the elasticity of the perineum by taking advantage of the hormonal changes that loosen connective tissue in late pregnancy. It also encourages relaxation of the pelvic floor muscles when there is pressure as there will be during birth. The likelihood of avoiding an episiotomy or serious tear seems to be improved by perineal massage.

To avoid an episiotomy or serious tear, it may be helpful to massage the perineum daily for about six weeks before the due date. Because perineal massage is unusual and personal, some caregivers are not familiar with it. Some women or couples find it distasteful and will not try it. Others feel it is worthwhile if it can reduce the chances of having an episiotomy. Some find it enjoyable, especially after doing it for a while and learning to relax.

If vaginitis, herpes, or other vaginal problems exist, perineal massage could worsen or spread the condition.

Instructions to the Woman or Couple
for Perineal Massage

Either you or your partner can do the massage. The first few times, take a mirror and look at your perineum so you know what you are doing. Be sure your fingernails are short. If you or your partner has rough skin on your fingers, it might be more comfortable to wear disposable rubber gloves. Wash your hands before beginning.

Make yourself comfortable in a semisitting position, squatting against a wall, or standing with one foot raised and resting on tub, toilet or a chair.

1. Lubricate your fingers well with oil or water-soluble jelly. Some people recommend wheat germ oil, available at health food stores, because of its high vitamin E content, but other vegetable oils can also be used. Do not use baby oil, mineral oil or petroleum jelly. To avoid contaminating the oil, rather than dipping your hands in the oil, squirt the oil over your fingers.

2. Rub enough oil or jelly into the perineum to allow your fingers to move smoothly over the tissue and lower vaginal wall.

3. If you are doing the massage yourself, it is probably easiest to use your thumb. Your partner can use his index fingers. Place the fingers or thumb well inside the vagina (up to the second knuckle); move them upward along the sides of the vagina in a rhythmic U or sling-type movement. This movement will stretch the vaginal tissue, the muscles surrounding the vagina, and the skin of the perineum. You can also massage by rubbing the skin of the perineum between the thumb and forefinger (thumb on the inside, finger on the outside or vice versa). In the beginning, you will feel tight, but with time and practice, the tissue will relax and stretch.

4. Concentrate on relaxing your muscles as you feel the pressure. As you become comfortable massaging, increase the pressure just enough to make the perineum begin to sting from the stretching. (This same stinging sensation occurs as the baby's head is being born.)

5. Massage for about five minutes. If you have any questions after trying the massage, ask your caregiver.

Appendix B. Teaching the Squatting Position

Penny Simkin, R.P.T.

The squatting position for second stage is a common birthing posture in many cultures, especially those where squatting (as opposed to sitting) is the customary resting position. The position has many advantages, as described in Carr's chapter in this book.

The squatting position does not, however, come naturally to most Western women who have become accustomed to sitting on chairs during their lifetimes. Therefore, there is need to teach women the mechanics as well as the benefits of squatting, and to encourage them to use it during labor and birth, especially if there is delayed progress in descent or a fetal malposition.

Following are the key points to make when teaching squatting to pregnant women:

1. Begin practicing squatting as early as possible in pregnancy (or before).

2. The goals are to be able to squat for up to two minutes at a time in a stable squatting position, with weight equally distributed over the soles of both feet, and then to rise to standing without using your arms to pull or push up. This should be done about 10 times a day.

3. Standing with your feet spread comfortably apart (toes straight ahead or pointing out, as is comfortable) and keeping your heels on the floor, slowly lower yourself to a squatting position. Stay down for 2 minutes or until your circulation gets "tingly," your knees or your insteps hurt, or you develop other discomfort. Then arise, unassisted.

4. While squatting, practice shifting your weight from side to side, and into kneeling positions, first on one knee and then the other. This kind of movement may assist fetal rotation and descent in labor.

TROUBLESHOOTING AND PROBLEM SOLVING

1. If you cannot keep your heels flat:
   a. Spread your feet wider apart.
   b. Wear shoes with 1 to 2 inch heels.
   c. Place your heels on 1 to 2 inch books or blocks.
   d. Slide down to squatting with your back against a wall.
   e. Hold onto doorknobs on either side of a door, or to partner's hands, leaning back enough to maintain heels on floor.
   f. Practice often, progressing toward keeping heels flat.

2. If you cannot maintain your balance:
    a. Use wall or partner or hold onto furniture for support.
3. If you are unable to rise from squatting without using your hands:
    a. Practice half-squats and wall-sitting to increase thigh strength. Squat halfway and rise to standing 10 to 20 times a day, and/or lean with your back against a wall with knees bent to a half-squat. Remain for 30 to 60 seconds at a time.
    b. Use assistance to get up while you build strength.
4. If your feet roll inward onto your insteps:
    a. Use same measures as with Number 1.
5. If you have pain in knees or hips:
    a. Determine the cause.
    b. If due to weakness, use measures for Number 3.
    c. If due to joint injury or arthritis, don't use squatting.
    d. If due simply to unfamiliarity with the position, begin squatting for short periods and gradually work up.
6. If you have pain in pubic symphysis (due to profound softening of the cartilage):
    a. Start with partial squats, lowering to the point where the pain begins. Then rise. It may improve with time, but if it does not, squatting may have to be abandoned.

With practice and with the motivation that comes when you know the potential benefits of squatting, you will be ready and able to use the position for comfort and/or progress in labor. During labor, it is desirable to avoid medications and interventions that interfere with or impede your ability to squat. It is also important to remain active throughout labor, changing positions both in and out of bed, using walking, hands-and-knees, sitting, standing and lying down on your side, in addition to squatting. It is more difficult to squat after hours of laboring in bed than after remaining active.

Remember, therefore, that squatting is only one of many possible positions for second stage. However, because it provides some advantages not present in other positions, it behooves you to master the technique and use it, if necessary, in second stage labor.

Appendix C. Memo To Obstetric Staff

Penny Simkin, R.P.T.

Childbirth educators who teach spontaneous bearing down and freedom of maternal position in second stage frequently find that nurses and physicians do not support this during labor. This may be upsetting to the laboring woman and her partner. The lack of support for physiological management is usually due to the caregiver's misunderstanding or lack of information. The following "memo" concisely explains the physiological second stage techniques. Childbirth educators can give a copy to each pregnant student to show to and discuss with her physician or midwife in advance. In addition, the memo can be shared with the nurses on arrival at the hospital. The memo may spare the woman or her partner having to explain these somewhat complex concepts while in labor.

The childbirth educator should also try to provide inservice education on these techniques at local hospitals.

FROM:___(Childbirth Educator's name)___ PHONE:_____

DESCRIPTION OF SECOND STAGE TECHNIQUES

This letter has been prepared to explain how *(Woman's name)* will be working during the second stage if she has no anesthesia. The techniques she has been taught are new and may be somewhat different from what you are most familiar with.

The differences you may notice are:

1. Mother's position: She has been encouraged to take whatever position is most comfortable to her and to vary her position during second stage until delivery: semi-sitting, sitting, sidelying, hands-and-knees, standing, squatting, etc. She has been discouraged from using the lithotomy or any supine position during descent of the baby, and for delivery unless and until forceps, vacuum extractor or episiotomy become necessary.

2. Bearing down efforts: Rather than prolonged breathholding and bearing down throughout the contractions, her bearing down and breathholding efforts will be spontaneous and in response to the strength and duration of her urge to push. Bearing down will be for a shorter period (5 to 6 seconds) than is usually encouraged. There may be several moments between these bearing down efforts during which she will breathe without pushing. Early in second stage she may have little or no impulse to bear down. This lull or "latent phase" passes within 10 to 20 minutes and her urge to push then increases.

3. Pelvic floor relaxation: This is of extreme importance.

YOU CAN HELP THE MOTHER BY:

1) suggesting that she try changing position if progress is slow, especially to gravity-enhancing positions;

2) reminding her to bear down with her urge, and not to push unless she has an urge;

3) reminding her to "let go" thereby relaxing the pelvic floor;

4) applying hot compresses to the perineum to encourage relaxation;

5) and, if spontaneous bearing down and changing position do not result in progress, asking her to bear down longer and more forcefully.

RATIONALE

Prolonged breathholding, straining and bearing down, and the supine position are associated with fetal hypoxia and acidosis, maternal hypotension, and/or too rapid distention of the vaginal tissues, increasing the possibility of lacerations and the need for episiotomy.

Spontaneous bearing down efforts with breathing between results in better oxygenation of the fetus and gradual distention of the vagina. Second stage may last longer than with prolonged bearing down and breathholding, but the fetus usually remains in good condition throughout.

Varying the position according to the mother's choice may assist fetal descent and rotation, especially in prolonged second stages.

The mother has discussed the above with her physician or midwife and has his/her approval.

REFERENCES

1. The normal second stage of labour: a plea for reform in its conduct. Beynon CL. J Obstet Gynaecol Br Commonw 64(6):815-820, 1957. (Reprinted in this volume.)

2. The influence of maternal bearing down efforts during second stage on fetal well-being. Caldeyro-Barcia R. Birth Fam J 6(1):Spring 79. (Reprinted in this volume.)

3. Alternative positions for childbirth - Part II: second stage of labor. Roberts J. J Nurs Midwif 25(5):Sep/Oct 80.

4. Influence of the duration of second stage labor on perinatal outcome and puerperal morbidity. Cohen WR. Obstet Gynecol 49(3):Mar 77.

5. Obstetric delivery today: for better or worse? Dunn PM. Lancet:790-93, 10 April 76.

Appendix D. Perineal Massage and Hot Compresses in Second Stage Labor

Lesley Weatherston, M.Sc., R.N., S.C.M.(U.K.)
Anne Robertson, R.N., S.C.M.

1. PURPOSE
   a. To stretch the perineum
   b. To avoid lacerations and need for episiotomy
   c. To relieve burning sensation as perineum stretches
2. POLICY
   a. Procedure is performed in 2nd stage of labor
   b. The nurse will wear gloves
3. OBJECTIVES
   a. To reduce resistance on perineal floor
   b. To achieve a thin and fully stretched perineum
   c. To reduce trauma to perineum
   d. To reduce the likelihood of Episiotomy 40-50%
4. MATERIALS
   a. Olive oil in squeeze bottle (or lubrication)
   b. Gloves
   c. Hot water and cloths (or gauze squares)
5. PROCEDURES

Action	Rationale
a. Start when head is just visible.	
b. Do only between contractions.	It does not interfere with her efforts to feel through the contraction.
c. Work on internal muscle bands, the best strokes are either smooth, full range ones following the sweep of the entire band or else direct, deep ball of fingers pressure penetrations on the tightest areas.	Both are good -- the first thins out and stretches, the second breaks up and unknots tension.
d. Half circular strokes in "U" shape on the perineum itself between points "three and nine o'clock" alternated with finger inside thumb outside, grasp-and pull outward thinning strokes.	To prevent tearing and need for episiotomy.
e. Very hot compress (almost difficult to touch) may be applied to perineum as head descends further.	To ease the burning sensation; increase circulation; relax perineum.

f. Where burning is experienced (Dick-Read's "Ring of Fire") instruct mother to stop pushing, depending of course, on fetal condition.

This is usually the point where internal lacerations start.

g. As the head is crowning, ask the mother to pant.

This gives the perineum extra time to stretch.

h. With one hand on the perineum push upward and inward, and with the other hand keep the head flexed by placing fingers over the occiput downward pressure.

This creates more slack in the tissue, and eases baby's head over the perineum.

i. Watch perineum carefully -- be sure it stays pink and is not pulled too taut. Watch for it turning white with strain, if so, stop patient pushing and repeat compresses.

Signs of imminent laceration.

6. DOCUMENTATION
    a. Partogram
    b. Interprofessional progress notes

REFERENCES

1. Saxell L. "Preventing Tears in Second Stage," unpublished, 1983.
2. Davis E. Heart and Hands: A Guide to Midwifery. New Mexico, John Muir Publications, 1981.

Author Index

Vasicka A, 21
Vedam S, 113

Walters R, 3, 20, 88, 108
Weatherston, Lesley, 121
Whalley, Janet, 115
Watson BP, 28, 32
Watson P, 86
Wertz DC, 88
Wertz RW, 88
Wessel H, 19
Wilkins M, 87
Wodell DA, 20
Wood C, 88

Yeates DA, 21, 113

Zilkoski M, 113

Subject Index

Abdominal muscles, 38
Adductors, 40
Adrenalin, 71, 73
Ambulation 51, 62, 72
Anal sphincter, 65, 110
Analgesia
  appropriate use of, 63, 73
  disadvantages of, 59, 63, 73
  for episiotomy, 64, 66
  postpartum, 66
Anesthesia
  advantages of, 12, 73
  disadvantages of, 12, 73
  for episiotomy, 91, 110
Anus, 33, 37, 99
Aorta, compression of, 11, 49,
  52, 54
Apgar scores, 12, 109, 112
Asymmetrical position, see
  Maternal positions

Back massage, 50
Back pain, 50, 52, 53
"Battering ram," fetal head
  as, 10
Bearing-down effort
  premature, 24, 27
  prolonged
    appropriate use of, 19, 29
    clinical trial of, 112
    closure of glottis during,
    43, 46-48
    compared with spontaneous,
    44-48, 112
    definition of, 43
    effects on fetus, 12, 44,
    46-48, 57, 74, 120
    effects on mother, 27-29,
    46-47, 74, 120
    historical perspective, 23
  spontaneous
    description of, 16, 119
    diagram of, 43
    clinical trial of, 112
    effects on fetus, 4, 10-
    11, 44, 46, 47-48, 120
    effects on mother, 10-11
    optimal duration, 44, 47,
    74, 119

    role of lateral abdominal
    muscles, 38
    "surges" in uterine
    contractility, 16
    variation among
    contractions, 24
    vocalization with, 16
  uncoached
    advantages of, 39
    clinical trial of, 26-27
    illustration, 31
    length of second stage,
    24-26
    suggestions for birth
    attendant, 24, 58
Bearing-down reflex, 12-13
Birth
  cultural determinants of,
  34-35
  historical trends in, 9-12
  prenatal education for, 71
  role of instinct in, 34-35
Birth attendants, vii, 2, 57
Birth canal, 27-29
Birth centers, episiotomy rate
  for, 86
Birthing stool, 51
Bladder, 33, 37
Bladder fascia, 28
Bladder supports, 28-29
Blood loss, 91, 93, 98
Body image, 103-108
Breastfeeding, 58, 104
Breathholding, prolonged, 4,
  12, 47, 112
"Breathing the baby out," 11
Breech delivery, 53, 61, 72,
  90, 99
Burning sensation and
  crowning, 17, 59, 74,
  116, 121, 122

Cardinal movements, 12
Catecholamines
  fetal, 10, 13
  maternal, 4
Cervical ligaments,
  transverse, 27
  illustration, 31

comfort measures for, 66, 106

comparison of episiotomy and laceration, 103-104, 109-110

table of, 104

effect on breastfeeding, 97,104

effect on intercourse, 93-94, 100, 104-109

effect on postpartum recovery, 93, 97, 110

rate of, 85

sources of, 2, 89, 99-100, 108

Episiotomy rate

optimal, 86

reasons for increase, 1, 57, 90

with squatting position, 111

Episiotomy repair

analgesia for, 66

compared to repair of laceration, 93, 110

controversies over, 82

difficulties with, 2, 92, 98, 106

doctors' attitudes towards, 105

"Husband's stitch," 106

intercourse following, 66

maternal reactions to, 92

performed by, 65, 92

postpartum care, 66, 99

procedure for, 65-66, 99

illustration, 101-102

suture materials for, 65

timing of, 92

wound breakdown, 65-66, 93

wound granulation, 2, 66

wound infection, 2, 85, 104, 110

wound inspection, 65

Exercise and episiotomy, 110

Expulsion, see Second stage of labor, phases of descent, transition

Ferguson reflex, 12-13

Fetal acidosis, 47-48

Fetal brain damage, 84

Fetal distress, 13-14

iatrogenic, 11, 57

Fetal heart rate patterns

bradycardia, 12, 14

decelerations, 12, 13, 44, 46, 74

definition of normal, 72

Fetal hypoxia, 12, 46-48, 71, 84, 120

Fetal malposition, positions for, 117

Fetal monitoring, electronic, 44, 72

Fetal rotation, positions for, 117

Fetal scalp blood pH, 12

Fetal well-being, indices of, 12

First stage of labor, 23, 62, 72-73

Forceps delivery, 1, 2, 4, 12, 25, 28-29, 61, 90, 110

Forceps rotation, 99

Fourchette, 63, 64, 99

"Genese de l'homme ecologique," Michel Odent, 35

"Gentle birth," 11

Glottis, 43, 74

Glutei, 40

Hands-and-knees position, see Maternal positions

Hematoma, 110

Hemorrhage, 2, 13

Hemorrhoids, 53, 98, 99

Hormones, stress, see Catecholamines

"Husband's stitch," 106

Hypotension

maternal iatrogenic, 11

supine, 4, 12

Imagery, 18

Infection, see Episiotomy repair, wound infection

Informed consent, 64

Intercourse

pelvic floor during, 34, 36

postpartum, 105-108, 109, 110

women's reactions to, 73-74
supported squat
advantages of, 50, 51
instructions for, 51
standing, 119
advantages of, 50
instructions for, 51
miscellaneous positions
hands-and-knees, 111, 119
advantages of, 53, 75
indications for, 39, 53
instructions for, 54
kneeling
advantages of, 53, 117
instructions for, 54
sitting, 119
definition of, 53
disadvantages of, 53
instructions for, 53-54, 72
Maternal positions for
intercourse, 105, 107-108
Maternal risk status, 72
Medical care, economic
considerations of
providers, vii
Medications, see Analgesia;
Anesthesia
"The Midline Episiotomy," Y.
Gordon, 33
Morphine, 9
Mortality rates, maternal, due
to episiotomy, 85

National Childbirth Trust
(N.C.T), vii, viii, 1,
103
Necrotizing fasciitis, 85
Newton's Law of Gravity, 49

Occiput posterior, 50, 61, 99
Oils, see Lubricants
Orgasm, 34, 36
Our Bodies, Ourselves, Boston
Women's Health Book
Collective, 80
Oxytocin, 13

Pain, see Back pain;

Dyspareunia; Episiotomy
pain; Labor pain
Pain relief
non-pharmacologic
techniques, 73
pharmacologic techniques,
see Analgesia; Anesthesia
Partogram, 2, 122
Parity, changes in, 81
Pelvic diameters, 49-50
Pelvic floor
analogy to "figure 8," 33,
37
analogy to mouth, 39-40
factors inhibiting normal
function, 35-36
functions of, 33-34, 36-39
relaxation of
suggestions for birth
attendants, 59, 120
suggestions for teaching,
40
techniques for, 18, 39-40,
115-116, 121-122
Pelvic floor anatomy, 97
illustration, 100
Pelvic floor awareness
goals of, 33-34
in male, 37
reasons for poor, 35-36
suggestions for teaching,
37-42
"elevator exercise," 37-38
"Happy Birthday," 40
"pelvic floor smile," 40
Pelvic floor contractions,
iatrogenic, 59-60
Pelvic floor damage, 2, 90,
109-112
Pelvic floor exercises
prenatal, 33-34, 37-42, 62,
70
postpartum, 41-42, 106
Pelvic floor relaxation, 84-85
Pelvic floor tone
postpartum recovery, 41-42,
77
suggestions for checking,
40-41
Pelvic inlet, 27
Pelvic "mouldability," 49-50

-131-